SLEEP STRATEGY BOOTCAMP – 28 DAYS TO CURE YOUR INSOMNIA, FAST!

The 11 Hardcore Anti-Insomnia Strategies that Kept Me Sane over the Last 25 Years – Effectively Stop Sleep Problems Now!

By: Tony Strong

Dedication

For Jane, Seven & Soda

Message from the author

Thank you very much for purchasing this book. I hope you gain real value and it will help you overcome your sleep problems. I would be very happy to answer any questions if I can. My email address is **tonystrong@helpbytony.com**

I'm sorry, I no longer offer face to face or Skype sleep counselling services.

I would be very grateful if you could leave a review for this book – we self-published authors REALLY rely on reviews to sell for our publications.

Thank you!

Tony

Table Of Contents

Introduction

If you find yourself having difficulties falling or staying asleep on a regular basis, the first thing you should know is that you're not alone. In an age of abundance, convenience, and luxury, at least from a historical perspective, the one thing we seem to lack is quality sleep. In relatively recent times, insomnia seems to have expanded to become a societal problem with no semblance of exclusivity to any group. It affects people from all walks of life, all classes, genders, races – it simply does not discriminate anymore.

In general, one in three people will show at least some symptoms of insomnia. To give you a better idea of how far-reaching this problem has become, consider the following findings that we have thanks to many years of research.

- In the United States, one in four people is subjected to insomnia every year.

- Some 30% of adult Americans report having symptoms of insomnia.

- For 10% of American adults, insomnia is a serious, chronic problem.

- Insomnia is a major burden on the US economy as a whole, costing around $63 billion every year.

- The link between insomnia and depression is very pronounced, with 83% of people diagnosed with depression reporting symptoms of insomnia.

- Insomnia costs many lives every year in traffic, being a major factor contributing to automobile accidents.

- Pregnant women are particularly vulnerable, with 80% of them reporting symptoms of insomnia during pregnancy.

- The incidence of insomnia is at a rate of 27% and 20% for working women and men, respectively.

- Older folks are especially vulnerable to insomnia, especially if they are of poor health.

- While countless men all over the world suffer from insomnia, women's incidence is higher.

- Workers who work in shifts are also traditionally prone to insomnia.

These shocking statistics offer but a glimpse into how serious this problem is on a massive scale. There are quite a few identified sleep disorders out there, such as sleep apnea, narcolepsy, REM sleep behavior disorder (RBD), restless leg syndrome, and others, but insomnia is the most common such disorder by far.

What is insomnia really, though? First and

foremost, if you find it difficult to fall asleep one night, then that's certainly no cause for alarm. The day's events, the anticipation of tomorrow, or a very temporary source of stress can make all of us toss and turn every now and then. Furthermore, our sleep patterns change throughout our lives, and that's natural. With age, for instance, your sleep requirements might become lower. It is your body that knows best how much sleep you need.

Insomnia is a recurring or outright chronic inability to fall or stay asleep. Simply put, it doesn't seem to go away and, what's more, its effects will begin creeping into our daily lives, affecting us in a million different ways. Insomnia can manifest in different patterns between different folks. Some insomniacs just can't fall asleep or sleep enough. Some will wake up in the middle of the night and be unable to go back to sleep for hours, effectively ruining their next day. The common denominator, however, is being tired and getting next to nothing out of your sleep, even if you do manage to doze off.

Waking up and feeling tired is just one in a million complications that can arise from insomnia, though. Those complications are, of course, almost always health-related, which drags along a whole bundle of other issues. This is one of the reasons why insomnia costs the economy so much. Because of it, people take more time off, they miss work, they get sick and ramp up insurance costs, et cetera. The market for products – mainly pharmaceuticals – which are used to treat symptoms of insomnia is itself expected to be worth around $4 billion by 2021. In all, just to list and explain all the problems that arise from not getting enough sleep would require a book of its own.

This book, however, is about solutions. It will take you on the important journey through the 11 steps or techniques of my Sleep Strategy Boot Camp process, which will help you in overcoming insomnia. Through this book, you will be taken on a breakthrough from your current situation to a renewed ability to get a good night's rest, which will demonstrate that your sleep problems can and will be solved.

You will find that some of my solutions are very straightforward and easy to implement. However, others will entail a lot of work and, most importantly, a rewiring of some of your habits, which can often be the hardest part. Many insomniacs have gotten to their dreadful position because of poor sleeping habits, so although hard, the part about habits is often necessary. The recommendations that you will find in this book are what I have built a sleep consultancy business on, though, and I now want to get this information across to a wider audience.

During my business venture, I have found that insomnia is an affliction with limitless reach, as it has brought many national and international clients to me over the years. For twenty years, I have been an NLP practitioner and consultant, specializing in sleep disorders during that entire time. My solutions are built around the goal of bringing balance back into the life of the reader, and they do so in a natural, drug-free manner. As everyone is different and insomnia can have a wide range of causes, this book will address the problem from many different angles. This means that you'll be presented with numerous alternative solutions, each offering a different approach relative to the cause but also the degree of the issue. It is a holistic approach and a step-by-step guide that will take you on a natural route toward a good night's rest.

On average, we spend around one-third of our lives asleep. As counterintuitive as it might seem in our contemporary society, which often gets its priorities wrong, sleep is one of the most important things you will do in life. It can't be overstated how profoundly the quality of your sleep is connected to your overall well-being. Consider the following examples, which will give you but a glimpse into how important and beneficial quality, natural sleep is.

- Seven to nine hours of uninterrupted, sound sleep will play an integral role in keeping your heart healthy

- A healthy sleeping pattern might reduce your risk of cancer.

- Your stress levels depend greatly on the quality and quantity of your sleep.

- Sleep reduces inflammation and the risk of future inflammation.

- Sleep makes you more alert in your daily life.

- Sleep is connected to your memory and the reliability thereof.

- Getting your sleep in order is important if you are trying to lose weight.

- A healthy sleeping routine keeps depression at bay, as well as countless other mental problems.

For more than twenty years, I've had experience with the stresses and turmoil of the corporate world. I was under a lot of pressure, often switching time zones, working nights, eating unhealthy, drinking, and relying on prescription drugs to keep my growing problems suppressed. To make matters worse, I was getting no exercise, and all of this had a profoundly negative impact on my sense of humor, outlook on life, and overall happiness. All the while, my career showed great promise and I was successful, but at a great price. I felt completely burned out, and my mental state seemed to deteriorate on a daily basis, with my sleep cycle getting ever-worse.

I sought medical help to deal with my problems, but this was to no avail. More often than not, I would just be given pills to treat the symptoms, not the cause. Certainly, the pills would usually shut me down like they are designed to, but I would wake up in the morning even more tired than I was. After a while, my restless nights were no longer just my personal problem – the consequences began to affect my relationship, which didn't last.

I felt that my entire life was spiraling out of control until things culminated when I fell asleep at the wheel. The resulting accident injured nobody but me, but this was my wake-up call, my moment of clarity. I realized that this was a problem I had to tackle head-on and fast, and that no magic pill exists. Over the following period, I spoke to healthcare professionals, therapists, and even spiritual leaders. Each piece of advice I gathered was like a crucial piece of one great puzzle, and that puzzle became my accumulated knowledge on the intricacies and importance of quality sleep. Some advice I had received was easy to implement, but other steps required dedication and hard work, but all of it was necessary for getting me to where I am now.

By following the strategies I will present, you too will benefit from the information, just like my many clients and I have. Understand, though, that you must be ready to commit to this journey. Reading this book will be just half of the first step out of many that you will have to take. There will be hurdles to surmount, but if you persevere and follow these strategies, you will get there. All of my past clients have seen great success with these methods and their sleeping problems have been dealt with. Stay on track, and this will work for you as well.

Remember – most cases of insomnia result from bad sleeping habits, and habits are often acquired over prolonged periods of time. Correcting bad habits will take time as well. You, your mind, body, and spirit will come together as a team and, with me as your coach, we will see you through to a good night's rest as effectively and quickly as possible. The benefits you reap will depend on the amount of effort you put in, the requirement for which will depend on your individual case. However, it won't take long at all for you to see the value in your commitment to beating insomnia, especially after you have read through the book.

The vast majority of cases of failure on this journey are a result of not sticking with your program. Unfortunately, some folks who have spent years acquiring their insomnia and then even more years suffering its reign of terror will give up if they see no results within days. Usually, it can take around a month for your body and mind to start adapting to the new way, but, again, that can vary between different people. Our common objective is for you to arrive at a stage where every morning brings you a sense of revitalization and refreshment when you wake up.

One important thing to note is that you should always consult with your doctor first so as to see if your insomnia is caused by a physical, medical condition. Indeed, insomnia can be caused by disease, physical pain, and many other similar issues that must be dealt with accordingly, but these cases are by far a minority. More often than not, insomnia is the result of our habits, life choices, and lifestyle, in which case it's all about behavior. Seeing as you have come to the point of reading this book, it's safe to assume that you have already confirmed that to be your case.

A good night's rest is more than a right – it is a primordial need – and your time to seize that right for yourself is now. Make the decision to get to work, and stop being a prisoner of this terrible affliction forever. The solutions are right there, and all you have to do is step forward. Read on and you will find that you have the strength to change these things, in addition to learning the necessary information.

Chapter One: Your New Beginning – Soothing Your Savage Breast

The best step to start with would be a simple one, which is exactly what we will do in this first chapter. As you can probably guess by now, insomnia and stress feed into each other and make each other worse. A great way to start your journey toward recovery is to find a way to relax not just moments before bed but also during the evening. As it turns out, there have been studies that have found that certain types of music have the potential to help us fall asleep easier.

As a 17th-century English author, William Congreve, noted in his play, *The Mourning Bride,* "Music hath charms to soothe the savage breast, to soften rocks, or bend a knotted oak." This means that music has the power to soothe and transform even the most tormented of folks and change lives, and science has since backed up Congreve's claim.

The studies conducted on this topic have come in from all over the world through the years. What's particularly important is that researchers have found that music can help alleviate sleep problems among folks from all age groups, men and women alike. What's more, even those people suffering from serious mental health issues have been observed to sleep better by using music. Furthermore, it seems that music can help us fall asleep whether we are having temporary trouble dozing off or are suffering from chronic insomnia.

Choosing the Right Music

In general, the experiments conducted have focused on getting the participants to soothe themselves by listening to calming music for a certain period before going to bed, usually 45 minutes. As you can imagine, certain types of music work much better than others. Rhythm is particularly important, and the music that's around sixty beats per minute tends to work best. This also happens to be the range to which our heart rate usually drops as we are falling asleep, and the music seems to help in getting our body to that level. As such, the music with that particular rhythm will act as an outside influence to help tune you into sleeping mode, so to speak.

As you can imagine, this is why people usually turn to classical music for this purpose. Classical music is far from the only choice, however, even though it perhaps offers the largest pool of music suitable for insomniacs. In fact, there are now many pieces of music available on the Internet, which have been designed specifically to help people sleep. Of course, there are also other well-established genres that might offer some soothing, sleep-inducing music, such as jazz.

Apart from the rhythm being around 60 BPM, there are other characteristics to look for. For instance, songs that are merely instrumental are almost always a better choice than those with lyrics.

Song lyrics usually have at least a vague semblance of a theme or meaning, which encourages thoughts in the listener. Although lyrical songs can be soothing, you might find yourself focusing unwittingly on the lyrics and drifting into thoughts and analysis, and you never know where that might take your mind.

Furthermore, it's a good idea to avoid music that is overly familiar to you, especially songs or pieces that are tied to anything in your life, especially something negative. Many people tend to attach a lot of their experiences and feelings to specific pieces of music, and listening to these songs when we are alone with our thoughts in the evening can get our minds racing. Positive thoughts can be a problem just the same. Unfamiliar music comes with no strings attached, so it is your safest bet.

Another thing to note is that just because a piece of music is slow and has adequate rhythm, it still might not be suitable. The music you choose must provide for some easy listening, and certain instruments are not really relaxing for most people even if the song is slow. Again, this is why most folks go with classical music to calm themselves in the evening.

However, with the advent and popularization of electronic music, especially these days, the options have never been more plentiful. As such, electronic music might be the best genre to look for your sleep music, especially if you're not too fond of classical. A great piece to start with, which sleep experts often refer to, would be a tune called "Weightless," by Marconi Union. Over the last couple of years, this track has often been referred to as the most soothing song in the world by many, and with good reason.

The song in question was designed and produced with total relaxation in mind. The rhythm and the tempo have been fine-tuned to soothe you into a state where your heart rate decreases and your brain reduces the production of stress hormones such as cortisol. As slow and relaxing as it is right from the get-go, "Weightless" gradually progresses to an even slower stage at around 50 BPM. The research that was done into the song's calming effects has found that the reductions in stress and anxiety for the listener are significant. Some researchers even advise against listening to this song in your car, especially on long drives, because of its potential to induce sleepiness.

Overall, it'll take a very quick Internet search for you to find that the number of options is potentially limitless. On top of that, there is a whole range of music out there designed specifically for the purpose of helping alleviate insomnia. As this approach to relaxing in the evening and inducting sleep becomes more popular, the number of choices will only grow.

Tips

First and foremost, some sleep coaches and consultants will recommend the use of things like headphones or earbuds to get maximally immersed in

19

the music. This might indeed work for you, but it's far from being the best solution. The good thing about them is that they really bring the music as close as possible, but these accessories can be uncomfortable and bother your body without you even noticing it. Relaxing is all about comfort, of course, so wearing headphones or earbuds will be the same as going to bed wearing your suit or a pair of jeans. What's more, earbuds that go deep into the ear can be dangerous while you're asleep, especially if you roll over.

Regular speakers are thus a much better choice. You can adjust the volume to how it suits your room layout and just go to bed as you would with a TV. Better yet, it's also possible to get pillow speakers, which do exactly what you would expect them to. You can buy the speakers themselves or look online for music pillows already equipped with the speakers. That being said, there are also headphones out there that are designed for listening to music and dozing off. Whether or not you want to invest in something like that is entirely up to you, but the important thing is to be as comfortable as possible.

You should also understand that the music that works best for someone else might end up having less of an effect on you. The general guidelines we have covered thus far will definitely apply, but there are always slight variations among the many musical pieces that fit the criteria. Depending on your mentality and the scope of your sleeping problem, these variations can be the difference between success and failure with this   particular strategy.

Therefore, you should take some time to experiment with different composers, instruments, and the like. Something else that might help you make a more personalized experience is some of the apps that have been developed to help insomniacs. Among these, you will find ones that make it easier for you to gather sleep music and create your collection.

You also don't have to restrict yourself to music per se. The Internet is loaded with great collections of various natural, ambient sounds that can be used for relaxation. These are often long recordings that help people fill their indoor spaces with the sounds of forests, rain, wind, or anything else they find soothing but are lacking in city life.

Furthermore and if possible, it's a good idea to use a timer to make sure that the music is turned off after a while. During certain stages of your sleep, you might be more prone to waking up even to sounds that relaxed you to begin with. Some people fall asleep very quickly, so they can time their music relaxation to last a mere fifteen minutes. People who struggle to fall asleep, however, should start with a wider window. You can try setting the timer to one hour at first and then adjust accordingly in the days to come. Again, certain apps can help you a whole lot in this regard.

Another thing to look out for are the conditions in your bedroom, particularly the air and the temperature. Try to have as much fresh air in there as possible by airing the place out before bedtime. Also, if it's too hot, it'll be difficult to relax since your body will be too busy trying to keep itself cool. The cooler the temperature the better you'll sleep, as long as you're not freezing, of course. The quality of the air you breathe can also be improved with various devices that can regulate all sorts of things including humidity, which should be kept at bay.

You should also never underestimate the ability of an uncomfortable bed to get in the way of your relaxation and sleep. Something that many folks don't consider is that a mattress should never be too soft. Certainly, it shouldn't be as hard as concrete either, but if your mattress gives in way too much, it might be a good idea to invest in a firmer, more comfortable one.

Soft beds can affect your back, neck, and many other areas that are prone to discomfort. Beds tend to get too soft as time goes by, but there are many other problems with old mattresses. Over the years, a mattress will accumulate all kinds of things such as dust, mites, dead skin, and sweat. All of these materials will make the mattress less porous and more difficult to keep cool, which can cause a lot of discomfort. If you've been using the same mattress for years, its replacement is a great place to start your journey to beating insomnia.

Creating Your Routine

To relax your body and mind as much as possible in the time leading up to sleep, it's a good idea to form a sort of routine for yourself. There's a lot of things you can do other than listen to music as a way of soothing yourself enough to doze off, and we'll cover some of these steps in much more detail as we proceed through the book.

For now, we'll take a look at a few general tips that might come in handy and go very well with calming music. Firstly, it's always a good idea to begin your evening routine with a soothing drink to calm your nerves instead of having a huge meal, and that doesn't mean a glass of whiskey. There are certain herbal teas that are known to reduce anxiety and make people sleep better, such as chamomile and valerian. Tart cherry juice is also an excellent choice. You can also use these beverages to help as a healthy substitute and alternative if you are trying to ditch coffee.

Another great addition to a relaxing evening routine is reading a book. Ideally, it shouldn't be difficult or heavy literature that'll make your brain hurt, but the most important thing is that it's a good old paperback book. We'll go into the reasons in more detail later, but distancing yourself from digital screens for a couple of hours before bed is highly recommended, as these can interfere with your sleep.

And so, instead of going directly to bed, you should take these couple of hours to remove the daily clutter from your mind and relax. Prepare a natural,

23

sedating drink, play some soothing music, pick up a book, and you will have the makings of an excellent routine.

By the time you're ready to doze off, the only remaining aspect of this routine should be the music. Try not to think about anything in particular, least of all your troubles or tomorrow's day. Your music can help you a lot in this regard, as you can focus on its rhythm and its instruments. Bringing these things into focus can drown out other mental noise and guide your mind into a semi-meditative state.

It's important to keep in mind that neither the music nor the rest of your new routine might yield results the very first night. It might take a while for your body to adjust but also for you to master the ability to let your mind relax, regardless of the music. Of course, there are many other things that you might find relaxing and should probably put into your routine. Take a long bath, take up a creative hobby, and try anything else that you think might calm your nerves.

Music and most other things we mentioned in this chapter will apply universally, but there's hardly a limit to how much you can personalize your evening routine. As we proceed, you will find many other tips and steps that might work very well with relaxing music and other evening activities. By the time we're through, you will see how many of these strategies feed into each other and work together as a holistic effort.

Chapter Two: Journalize Your Troubles Away

While music is bound to help in many cases, it's certainly not the only thing you can do to ease your mind and shift focus away from your worries. Many people carry a plethora of worries around from one day to the next, and these worries drag with them a whole range of negative feelings and stress. Such feelings and troubles have to be channeled and processed in a meaningful way. Otherwise, they can accumulate and fester if internalized, ending up as a major burden on your mind.

In many insomnia cases, even insomnia itself can become a source of anxiety and stress. After a while of torment, frustration, and hopelessness, you might get to a place where you can't stop thinking about your inability to fall asleep, which creates a terrible, vicious cycle. In order to fall asleep, your brain has to be calm and at ease, and saying that anxiety is the opposite of calm is an understatement. Stress is generally caused by a very real, inherent mechanism that all healthy human beings possess – their flight or fight response.

This mechanism kicks in when we feel that we are in danger and, in natural circumstances, it occurs when that danger is real, acting as an integral part of our survival mechanisms. In the hectic life in contemporary society, however, your brain can start interpreting all sorts of things as a threat, often chronically, leading to constant stress. Stress and anxiety are generally not the same, though, as similar as they might appear.

Stress is a reaction your body and mind have when they detect a perceived threat, which is usually a short-term factor. Since stress is completely natural, it's not always a bad thing. Stress can motivate and propel us forward, but it can also help us avoid dangerous situations. Stress becomes a very bad thing once it begins to affect your ability to concentrate, enjoy the things you used to, and fall asleep.

Anxiety, particularly in the context of mental health, is a disorder. This disorder is one that brings fear, which is often irrational and inexplicable, sometimes stemming from an unidentified source. Anxiety can be a result of stress but also trauma. One of the most important distinctions between stress and anxiety is that stress is supposed to cease once a perceived threat has been removed or dealt with. Anxiety, however, tends to be chronic, persistent, unpredictable, and very difficult to deal with. This feeling of unease and worry can manifest in a lot of physical ways apart from just insomnia. Anxiety has been known to impair people's ability to eat, focus, socialize, communicate, derive joy from their favorite activities, and much else.

Symptoms of Anxiety and Stress

As similar as they might be, it's certainly possible to tell which of the two problems you're experiencing if you know what to look for. Many of the symptoms are shared between stress and anxiety, but some are specific to the respective problem. Still, prolonged stress and anxiety alike can lead to a number of additional complications with implications for your overall health.

When it comes to stress, we can all tell when we're experiencing it in a given situation, as our reaction to stressful situations is fairly self-explanatory. When we're stressed out, we get tense, our palms sweat, our heart rate kicks up, et cetera. However, when you are experiencing too much stress and too frequently in a chronic manner, the consequences can be far-reaching. Apart from sleep problems, of course, you can end up suffering from frequent headaches, back pain, neck pain, fainting, dizziness, loss of appetite, constant muscle tension, forgetfulness, diminished sexual drive, poor concentration, gastrointestinal problems, and much else.

Stress can also have a dramatic impact on your immune system, which can lead to frequent illnesses and infections of all kinds. The truly terrible thing is that insomnia too can cause most of the issues we just mentioned, so a combination of chronic stress and a lack of sleep can be lethal. Stress also makes you irritable, which makes it difficult to perform at work,

27

communicate with people, or maintain personal relationships.

If stress is consuming your daily life, then that's something you will have to deal with. Apart from what we covered in the previous chapter, we will go over many other ways to deal with stress as we go along. One of the most common and simplest ways to cope with stress is controlled, deep breathing. Take at least a couple of seconds to fill your lungs with air. Then, hold it in for the same amount of time and, finally, exhale over a couple of seconds as well. This is a simple and immediate way to alleviate a stress attack for the time being, but it's often not the long-term solution.

When it comes to anxiety, it can torment you in many of the same ways, but the markings of an actual disorder are more pronounced. When you have an anxiety disorder, it's not uncommon for it to attack for seemingly no reason. This problem is usually characterized by excessive or outright obsessive worrying and a deep feeling of anxiety. If you experience this on a majority of your days for at least six months, it might be generalized anxiety disorder.

There are multiple kinds of anxiety disorders, but they all generally revolve around disproportionate outbursts of stress, fear, and worry even over trivial things. Take social anxiety for example. People who suffer from this disorder tend to get unreasonably stressed out in social situations even if there is no danger of any kind involved.

Needless to say, anxiety disorders can have a dramatic effect on your ability to sleep. Physically, anxiety can manifest in many ways. Similarly to stress, it can cause sweating, irritability, fatigue, rapid heart rate, muscle tension, shaking. There can also be shortness of breath, chest pain, a lack of concentration or outright mental block, overreactions of all kinds, stomachache, headache, and other issues.

Anxiety can suck all the joy right out of your life and make every day feel like hard labor. The disrupted sleep is just one out of many problems that this disorder can cause, and it's definitely something that needs to be dealt with. Anxiety can be a deep-rooted, serious condition in some cases, so it can often require psychotherapy or even medication. Nonetheless, there are many other things you can do to help yourself feel better and let go of some of your worries.

Managing Negative Thoughts and Feelings

The first step is to learn how to manage negative thoughts and emotions. Everyone experiences these negative responses from time to time and it's only natural, but not everyone processes that input the right way.

One of the worst things you can do is dwell on negative thoughts and allow them to grow bigger and heavier. We can't help but feel emotions and negative thoughts will occur when something is bothering us, but obsessing over such thoughts is essentially a choice. Instead of indulging in negativity and letting it take over, you should focus on healthy, productive things. One of the most common causes of recurring negative thoughts and feelings are traumatic or greatly disappointing events. When something that happens gets you down, the best thing to do is introduce lifestyle changes, many of which we'll cover as we proceed through this book.

The important thing is to try and identify the source of your negative thoughts and feelings. More often than not, it shouldn't be too difficult to do that, but sometimes the things that bother us can be more subtle. When it comes to anxiety, for instance, avoidance is generally the wrong thing to do. If normal things like social situations or conversations with certain people in your life give you anxiety, avoiding these things as a means of escape is likely to make the problem worse. The solution in such cases is to tackle the problem head-on, which can require counseling and other steps. At the very least, you'll sleep better knowing that you are working on your problems instead of aimlessly obsessing over them and worrying.

However, as you've learned by now, just because you sometimes worry or a few negative thoughts intrude on your mind doesn't mean that you have a full-fledged anxiety disorder. The first step toward dealing with your emotions better is to understand that they are simply data and information. Your emotions and intruding thoughts are not something to be eliminated but listened to. If you try to think about your worries objectively and with self-compassion, you will usually identify the problem much easier. You are the only person who can get to the root of the problem and understand what's worrying you and why. Counseling can help, but even then, it's you who has to open up and talk about your problems.

A lot of what you feel is also in the way you perceive things. Something that has you worried a whole lot would perhaps cause much less stress to someone else because the perspective is different. Failure or the fear of it, for instance, is a common cause of stress and worry for people, yet some seem to be bothered very little by it. However, failure is also a great example of how a mere change in perspective can help so much. Instead of looking at failure as the death of your prospects, you should focus on what you can learn from it each time before you give it another shot. Failure is just one example, of course, but the important thing to remember is that perspective really can be everything.

Another important step in dealing with the negativity in your mind is to find outlets. Creative endeavors, exercise, a simple hobby, and much else can come in handy. These things will help you focus on healthy aspects of life and might also improve your health and shape, which is always a great way of combating stress. It's important to treat yourself well and indulge in self-care and improvement. You'll find plenty of ways to do that throughout this book, but it all has to start with your own decision and willingness to get better. It's unfortunate, but it can be very difficult to let go of our worries and stop obsessing over them when we're alone with our thoughts at night. In fact, sometimes we don't want to give these thoughts up on a subconscious level, but we have to.

Journals and Lists

Externalizing the feelings and thoughts that bother you through a journal or a similar outlet can be a great help in dealing with your problems. This simple solution is often overlooked because of that simplicity, but writing things down is severely underrated.

You can start with a plain old diary or journal where you will log the day's events, including everything that went wrong and right. If a day isn't particularly eventful, you can try to note your thoughts, both negative and positive. Once you put all of these things down on paper and have them sit in front of you, you will look at them differently. It will be easier to sort your thoughts out and shift your focus to what was good about your day. You shouldn't shy away from writing down even the most mundane of things. Once you have done this for a while, you'll see it for yourself, but even seemingly irrelevant things can look different when written down.

When it comes to dealing with the sources of your stress, writing a list can be very helpful. You should list all of your stressors in daily life, whether they stem from work, family life, or anywhere else. It will thus be easier for you to categorize these problems and look at them objectively. When you are unsure why you were stressed or anxious, it's a good idea to just list all of the situations that made you anxious that day. Looking at these incidents objectively can help you get to the bottom of the problem.

What's also interesting and perhaps surprising is that recent studies have shown that simple to-do lists can help us fall asleep. If you are the kind of person who likes to write down a to-do list in the morning, you might want to consider doing that in the evening instead. The studies done on this topic stem from a hypothesis that the act of writing down a to-do list for tomorrow's tasks might be a good way to alleviate some of the worries on our minds. As such, this might be an activity that you would want to introduce into your evening routine while you're relaxing before going to sleep.

You can try to go for two days in advance when writing the list, but you can also take it a lot further than that. For instance, writing down your long-term goals, dreams, and wishes in life might also have a soothing, therapeutic effect in the evening.

As simplistic as this might seem, it can definitely be one of those small, relaxing activities that help occupy and then ease our minds in the evening hours. You can also experiment and try writing down anything else that might be weighing on your mind. It doesn't have to be a long session either. You should simply keep a notepad or journal and a pen on your nightstand and take five minutes every evening to dump some of your mind's troublesome contents onto the paper.

Chapter Three: Late to Bed, Early to Rise

As you can imagine, the way you go to bed, so to speak, has a lot to do with the quality of your sleep, as well as the way you get up in the morning. There are many bad habits that plague both our mornings and evenings nowadays, and they can often disrupt our sleep cycle.

Back in the old-old days when rural and agricultural lifestyles were the norm, daily life exerted a lot of physical energy every single day. Usually, folks who had to plow their fields and tend to their livestock or work around their farms would be all but exhausted by the evening. On top of that, there wasn't much in the way of distraction and entertainment to keep them up late. Their sleep cycles were usually very natural as long as they were healthy, and they would rise early and rested.

Nowadays, the majority of our jobs require no meaningful physical activity at all and the energy we exert is mostly in brainpower. Sometimes, however, we don't really get to grind our brains much at work either. Combined with a lack of exercise, this accumulated energy can make it incredibly difficult to relax and set in for bedtime until at least midnight.

Forcibly Adjusting Your Internal Clock

As a part of many behavioral therapy programs, therapists will often use something called sleep restriction therapy for one or two sessions. The trouble with some insomniacs who keep waking up during the night and losing hours of sleep is that they will sometimes try to make up for it by staying in bed longer. This upsets the sleep cycle even further and can make it even more difficult to fall asleep the following night.

The idea behind sleep restriction therapy is to prevent that by force through the designation of a strict time window that the patient can spend in bed. Naps are also severely restricted or eliminated, all in the interest of gradually adjusting your brain and body to fall asleep at the required time. If your brain just refuses to fall asleep at that designated time, then the going will get quite tough at first. You might end up very sleep deprived for days, which is one of the main concerns when it comes to this method of therapy. It's especially problematic for workers who need to be alert and focused on their job lest they put someone else's life in jeopardy.

Nonetheless, sleep restriction therapy might indeed reduce the time it takes you to fall asleep, but it's also likely to improve the quality and efficiency of the sleep you get. That's after your body has finally gotten accustomed to the change after a sometimes turbulent adjustment period.

If it's safe for you and your line of work, you can certainly give sleep restriction a try. Take note of how many hours you spend asleep during the night, and then restrict the time you spend in bed down to that exact time. This means no more discounting the time you spend lying in bed before and after you sleep. If you tend to get six hours of shuteye, no matter how unstable it is, then that's the time you should spend in your bed starting at the most suitable time of the evening.

Things are likely to get much worse from that point onward until you begin to readjust. This therapy generally spans a period of four weeks, at which point you should start to experience a noticeable difference in how fast you fall asleep and how rested you feel in the morning. What's also worth mentioning is that, as a rule of thumb, you shouldn't make your bedtime shorter than five hours even if that is the amount of time you generally get to sleep.

While some insomnia treatment centers or sleep coaches might use sleep restriction therapy and variations thereof as their main program, you can do it differently. Sleep restriction can be just one of many attempted strategies in an arsenal of skills that can be used as parts of a holistic, all-encompassing approach that tackles the problem from all sides. This is exactly our objective in this book, putting as many eggs into as many different baskets as possible.

Apart from just boosting your daytime drowsiness even further and making you less alert, sleep deprivation might boost the symptoms of certain mental disorders such as bipolarity. For some people such as those who have a severe bipolar disorder, sleep deprivation or any such strategy can turn into a nightmare, so it's not recommended.

Overall, combating your insomnia in this manner is a rather crude approach that might work, but you will learn soon enough that there are countless alternatives that are healthier and easier. Simpler routines, some dietary adjustments, and a regular, soothing evening ritual can do the trick for lots of insomniacs.

The Dos and Don'ts

There are countless smaller adjustments that you can make to the way you go to bed, sleep, and conduct yourself in the evening overall. There's also a bunch of that's not such a good idea.

You should generally avoid going to bed until you're at least moderately relaxed. You can use the preparation of your evening routine to take your mind off things and gradually relax as bedtime draws near. By the time you are under the covers, you will be hallway there and your sleep music should help you the rest of the way.

If you have trouble with sleep latency, or the time it takes to fall asleep, it's not a good idea to go to bed too early. You will only spend more time in the bed doing nothing or, worse yet, getting angry over your insomnia. Instead, you should greet your early onset of sleepiness while you're somewhere other than your bedroom. If you get to your bed already somewhat sleepy, the feeling of settling down and covering up can speed up the process.

Furthermore, while some people find the sound of their clock to be soothing and great for rocking them to sleep, insomniacs should probably avoid clocks. Obviously, the main association when thinking of a clock is time, and if you're listening to it ticking away while struggling to fall asleep, it can begin to demoralize you even further. Even more importantly, don't look at the clock either.

If you don't normally use alarms to wake you up, you might want to give them a try at least for a while. An alarm can help you get a grip on your sleep cycle and run some experiments to see how you feel waking up at different points in time. The important thing is that you get up fast and without hesitation once the alarm goes off in the morning. Don't snooze like so many people seem to enjoy nowadays.

Cutting your sleep up into little pieces while already struggling to maintain a good night's rest is the opposite of what you want to do. Snoozing can really interfere with the phases of your sleep and also make it more and more difficult to get up after each snooze, making you wake up particularly drowsy.

Next, if you already engage in some sort of daily exercise or are planning to get started, you should make sure that you exercise early in the morning, earlier in the day, or during the afternoon, but never too close to your bedtime. You should maintain at least three or so hours between an exercise routine and your desired shuteye time.

The morning is a particularly good time to exercise for insomniacs because physical activity early in the day can make you more alert and subdue the symptoms of drowsiness and exhaustion brought on by your insomnia.

You don't want to ingest too much fluid in the later hours of the day either, but there are certain drinks that folks have found beneficial for their sleep for centuries. One example is a glass of warm milk. You can try drinking a glass or mug of this milk in the evening, but you should be careful not to drink too much or make it too hot. Either scenario can upset your stomach and give you all sorts of trouble in the night.

These were a quick few pointers to help introduce you to the world of things that might affect your sleep positively and negatively. We'll elaborate more on this in our next section, but you should already have a solid idea of how complex sleep actually is and how much room there is for us to mess it all up.

Advice on Maintaining Sleep Hygiene

Something called sleep hygiene plays a big role in many forms of behavioral or combined therapy that are available out there. While it does touch upon some aspects of your personal hygiene, you shouldn't let the term fool you as sleep hygiene is about much more than taking a shower and equipping your bed with some clean linen.

Sleep hygiene is essentially a range of things that constitute good sleeping habits and promote quality sleep. If you go to bed whenever you please, drink a lot of coffee, or eat enormous meals before bedtime, you are indulging in very poor sleep hygiene. What follows are some of the main aspects of proper sleep hygiene, most of which we'll explore in more detail later on.

Good sleep hygiene dictates that you minimize your use of any and all stimulants or remove them from your life completely if possible. Nicotine, caffeine, alcohol, stimulating tea plants, and maybe even some of your prescription drugs can all stimulate your brain and keep you up at night. The closer you get to bedtime, the more you should avoid all of these. If you're having trouble sleeping, then most of your afternoon and especially evening hours should be stimulant-free.

Taking naps is definitely poor sleep hygiene, especially if you take them at random points in the day, for random durations, and whenever you get the faintest semblance of sleepiness. If you suffer from insomnia, then you will feel tired often during the day. Indulging in naps because of your drowsiness will only deepen the problem.

Furthermore, while the average sleep requirement for most adults is between seven and nine hours or so, it's ill-advised to try and force yourself to fit that mold. If you need to sleep a bit longer, you should try and accommodate yourself. On the other hand, just because you slept for fewer hours doesn't mean you can't be rested. Good sleep hygiene will improve the efficiency and quality of your sleep, which is generally more important than quantity.

It's not a particularly good idea to try and force yourself to sleep by just lying in bed for hours on end. This can lead to a lot of frustration and stress or even obsession over your insomnia, which only makes it worse. Instead, you should strive to take steps during the day that will include your likelihood of being sleepy in the evening.

Another step toward better sleep hygiene is the minimization of all potentially interfering stimuli in your sleeping environment. Of course, that doesn't include any stimulus that's there specifically to promote sleepiness, such as your sleep music as discussed in the first chapter. Your bedroom should be devoid of powerful smells, noises, and, most of all, strong lights, particularly white LED lights or blue light emissions from digital screens.

It's also in the interest of good sleep hygiene to keep your sleep scheduled and consistent. Going to bed and waking up at a similar time each day is ideal because it will reduce many of the internal fluctuations that occur when we sleep inconsistently.

This can be upsetting to numerous aspects of your health and biological processes, but especially the sleep cycle.

All of that should give you a solid introduction into what sleep hygiene as well as a taste of some of the changes you will have to introduce into your life if you are to get your sleep cycle back on track. Along the way, we will get into these and other recommended changes in more detail and also explain why certain habits are good or bad for sleep.

Chapter Four: Remove Harmful Substances

There are quite a few substances that have become part and parcel of modern living, which can be incredibly harmful not just to our ability to sleep but also overall health. Smoking and consumption of nicotine, for instance, are becoming less common and socially acceptable, but they are still all but common, in some places more than others.

Then there's one of our society's closest friends – caffeine. Our coffee habit has been the object of many studies looking for a range of different answers. When it comes to its impact on our lives and health, caffeine is not necessarily all bad, but it might be considered a mixed bag at times.

Of course, caffeine isn't anywhere near as problematic as alcohol, the abuse of which is on the rise in the United States, as well as a traditional and major problem in other parts of the world. The health implications of alcohol abuse are immense and, as you can imagine, this problem doesn't get along well with your ability to sleep.

There is also the matter of pharmaceuticals, among which sleeping pills are the most pertinent to our problem. Sleeping pills are definitely a checkered issue, as they might indeed be necessary and can help us at times, but they come dragging a whole range of potential problems.

In this chapter, we will take a more detailed look at these harmful substances and their relationship with our sleep cycle. The thing about certain substances such as caffeine is that they might not be particularly bad in moderation, but then again, there might be no real need for them either. This is especially true when you already have sleeping problems. Overall, eliminating these substances is bound to pay off in the long run as nothing can really compete with a clean body that relies only on itself instead of substances that provide a crutch to depend on.

Nicotine

It goes without saying that smoking is a blight that should befall none. Without getting into the five million different ways in which smoking can harm or kill you, it's worth pointing out that nicotine has implications for your sleep as well. Nicotine is a stimulating substance, so just because you're not getting it through cigarettes doesn't mean that it can't contribute to insomnia. Indeed, nicotine can be had in a number of ways nowadays, so if you use nicotine patches, chewing gum, or vape with an e-cig, all while having trouble sleeping, you will want to abandon these products and remove nicotine from your life altogether.

You shouldn't be too hard on yourself, though.

Quitting smoking is quite an achievement, but it's still true that nicotine substitutes can be something of a trap for many ex-smokers. Instead of helping you abandon your nicotine addiction altogether, substitutes can simply replace smoking and leave you addicted to a new product.

The impact that nicotine will have on sleep will vary from one person to the next and often depend on the degree of addiction. In general, the best thing to do is to eliminate nicotine altogether, of course, but what's especially problematic is when it's taken just before bed. Apart from its stimulating effects, nicotine might also make you crave more of it even when you're sleeping, which can wake you up. This is why it's better to be nicotine-free for as long as possible before bedtime, as you will have gotten over the initial craving by then.

Now, the stimulating effect can be next to non-existent for people who are heavily dependent on the substance because of their built-up tolerance. As with many other substance addictions, the effects of that substance can wear off over time and the cravings can become just a matter of keeping the substance's blood levels up.

Nicotine and especially smoking can cause a whole bunch of other problems, though. The very structure of a smoker's sleep is fragmented and abnormal; their sleep is more shallow and prone to interruption. Smokers also tend to take longer to fall asleep on average. All of these issues have been found to disappear for ex-smokers after a while of being nicotine-free.

On top of that, smoking significantly increases your risk of developing sleep apnea and snoring. Sleep apnea has the potential to be a very serious sleeping disorder, as it affects your breathing pattern while you sleep. It's one of the most common causes of waking up in the morning feeling tired, and it often goes hand-in-hand with insomnia.

These are only some of the sleep-related issues tied to smoking and nicotine in general. If you're a smoker, then there's no need to go into the endless reasons you should kick this habit, but now you know that it might be adding to your sleeping problems as well, which is additional motivation.

Alcohol

Nicotine and cigarettes might be highly addictive and devastating to your health, but smoking hardly has the potential to ruin families, destroy careers, and completely demolish all aspects of a person's life. Alcoholism can lead to so many problems that covering all of them would require a book series. However, you don't have to be a raging alcoholic for alcohol to disrupt your sleep and lead to a whole bunch of other health problems. Moderate habitual drinking, an addiction at its inception, and self-medicating with booze are all situations where quality sleep can suffer.

What's particularly tricky about alcohol is that

47

it often has a sedating effect and, of course, everyone knows that it can make a person doze off or pass out. Around 20% of adult Americans will end up using alcohol to fall asleep faster at least at some point. Don't be fooled, though, as alcohol is very likely to make insomnia worse over time, regardless of the temporary relief it might provide.

The trouble with alcohol is that it disrupts the structure of your sleep in that it makes it more difficult for you to enter the important REM stage of sleep. When this stage isn't reached or doesn't last long enough, your brain and body will not get the required rest. This happens because alcohol makes you fall into deep sleep much faster than is natural, making you spend less time in other states such as REM.

The real insidiousness is in the fact that using alcohol to fall asleep won't cause this problem right away. In fact, using booze as a sleeping pill might work rather well for a while, until it suddenly doesn't. Over time, you will become more likely to wake up during the night and you will feel less rested with each new morning. People will sometimes try to solve this problem by drinking more, which creates quite an obvious vicious cycle that leads to alcoholism.

Furthermore, drinking in the evening can also wake you up by forcing you to go to the bathroom in the middle of the night. Worse yet, alcohol dehydrates you through other means such as sweat, which can destabilize your sleep or get you to wake up with a headache. Just like smoking, alcohol also increases the possibility of snoring.

With all that said, alcohol is also a stimulant, as you well know if you drink. The same effect that gets you in a mood to party and have fun can leave your body and brain highly active even if you doze off. Alcohol can also wake you up during the process of leaving your system, whether through withdrawal or further disruption of your sleep structure. Of course, there's also the potential for a hangover. Even if it's a tiny hangover that you hardly even feel, things like your alertness and restfulness can still be affected.

Overall, alcohol is something that you need to remove or minimize as soon as possible if you have trouble sleeping. A glass of wine at an early dinner or a couple of beers with your friends obviously won't constitute problematic behavior, but you should avoid alcohol like the plague in the hours leading up to bedtime. Of course, your body can only benefit from the total elimination of alcohol from your life, but mere moderation can really do wonders and let you get the best of both worlds. Just remember that alcohol is not a solution to insomnia – quite the contrary.

Caffeine

When it comes to the enemies of sleep among substances, caffeine undoubtedly tops the chart. Being the most widely available and socially acceptable stimulant, caffeine is virtually everywhere, perhaps more now than ever before. Apart from coffee, you'll find caffeine in many places such as chocolate products, various teas, sodas, or energy drinks, which are essentially caffeine bombs.

Caffeine makes you more alert and energized, but it can also improve your concentration and offer a wide range of other benefits. As problematic as it can be for sleep, caffeine is far from being an evil substance. In fact, a lot of research in recent years and decades has outlined many benefits of moderate caffeine use, much to the pleasure of coffee drinkers everywhere. Nonetheless, there are also benefits to eliminating it from your life, so it's quite a mixed bag.

The important thing to note is that caffeine can stay in your system for quite a long time, sometimes up to eight hours. Not only does caffeine inhibit the production of sleep-inducing chemicals in your brain, but it can also increase your adrenaline. It takes a mere fifteen minutes for the effects of caffeine to kick in once it is ingested. On top of that, caffeine is physically addictive and some folks can develop quite a dependence on it. Even if you take what is considered a moderate daily intake of some three eight-ounce cups, containing around 250 milligrams of caffeine each, addiction is still highly likely.

Just like with the previous two substances, the first thing to do is to eliminate caffeine from the latter half of your day. You have no natural need for caffeine and it is little more than a mild, legal, worldwide stimulant. In fact, caffeine has all the makings of a drug. If you are dependent on caffeine, quitting it can result in headaches, fatigue, or even muscle pain. While uncomfortable, these withdrawal symptoms won't last very long, so quitting caffeine isn't the hardest habit to kick.

Despite some of its benefits, some studies have linked caffeine use to a range of problems such as increased anxiety, irritability, bladder sensitivity, and, of course, sleep problems. Overall, you can only benefit from removing caffeine from your life altogether. You can do it over a period of seven days where you will gradually reduce your daily intake to zero with the aim of minimizing your withdrawal symptoms. It might take a while, but you will eventually see many positive results of going caffeine-free. As for the morning coffee boost, you're better off replacing it with a healthy, natural alternative to get you up and going such as exercise.

Drugs

It goes without saying that doing drugs will do a lot worse than give you insomnia, but the problems certainly aren't limited to controlled substances. Legal drugs, prescription or otherwise, can be just as bad for your sleep cycle. What's more, doctors are often more than willing to give out prescriptions.

For many folks who suffer from insomnia, getting some sleeping pills is often the first thing that comes to mind, but pharmaceuticals come with a lot of strings attached. For one, sleeping pills are generally not a cure for insomnia. They are meant to help in the short-term and are in no way a substitute for a healthy, natural night of sleep.

Another problem is that insomnia is often accompanied by additional sleep disorders such as sleep apnea, and sleeping pills are essentially worthless in that regard. Their purpose is to induce sleepiness quickly and knock you out on demand. As you can probably gather, this doesn't address a single underlying issue. Your insomnia might be caused by anxiety, poor diet, poor sleeping habits, and all those other things, while a sleeping pill does little more than put you under for a few hours of what can sometimes be classified as artificial sleep.

If you have come to rely on these products for a long period of time, you should definitely stop. It's not just that the sleep you get from these pills is often not natural and restful, but your ability to sleep can come to depend on the pills, which is a very bad place to be in. Indeed, sleeping pills can be very addictive, particularly because you will quickly begin to build up a tolerance, so your body will require larger doses to get the same effect. Sleeping pills can also have daytime side-effects in the form of drowsiness, lack of focus, and other complications.

Sleeping pills are best used as a temporary crutch over a period of no more than a few months to help us through a rough time or as an additional help within other forms of therapy. Nonetheless, you are better off avoiding them altogether and resorting to healthier, natural strategies of combating your insomnia, plenty of which are contained in this book.

If you ever come to a situation where you truly feel like you have no choice but to use pharmaceutical assistance, then you should do so only after thorough counseling and evaluation by a sleep specialist. Those who use cognitive behavioral therapy to treat people's insomnia will usually have the best advice in this regard because their practice focuses on the exact opposite of using short-term pharmaceutical solutions to treat a long-term problem.

Chapter Five: Salute the Sun and Walk in Nature

As you have already gathered, so many of the problems that affect our sleep stem from the way we live in our post-industrial society. Urban living certainly has countless benefits and conveniences, but it's impossible to escape the fact that humans were made to walk the landscape, prowl the steppes, and navigate forests. Spending time in nature has immense health benefits, but going on a picnic once every two months just won't cut it.

Taking the time not just to visit a more natural environment but to also walk and engage in other activities is very important. That's just the beginning of the effort to reconnect with nature, though, as you also need to reconnect with your own, inner nature. This is why fitness programs and things like yoga are becoming increasingly popular throughout the Western world.

Exercise and Sleep

We will start with plain old exercise, which has a pretty intimate relationship with our sleep. At first glance, the matter at hand seems pretty obvious. Exercise will wear you out and make you tired, which equals drowsiness, which equals falling asleep quickly after your day is over. However, experts have conducted quite a bit of research into this topic over the years, and there are numerous particularities to discuss.

Firstly, some forms of exercise will be much more beneficial in beating insomnia than others. Aerobic exercise, for instance, is particularly useful because it makes one's cardiovascular system healthier, which reflects well on sleep quality. One of the studies on this was conducted by researchers at Northwestern University. The researchers used 23 middle-aged and older adults, most of whom were women. These participants reported living sedentary lives without much physical activity and they also reported trouble with their sleep.

They were divided into two groups with different exercise intensity. Both groups partook in the experiment for sixteen weeks and their exercise included stationary bicycles, walks, and treadmills. The researchers also put together a control group for the same period of time. This group only took part in mental exercise through recreation, education, and skill learning.

The study concluded a significant improvement in the sleep quality of the folks who exercised. The improvement was evaluated and confirmed by sleep experts who also noted that the participants reported feeling more vitality and being more upbeat in daily life, on top of being less sleepy and drowsy. These findings reaffirmed the research team's belief that drug-free treatments for insomnia were the best approach. This is especially important for middle-aged and older folks because they might already be on medication for other issues – medications that sleeping pills could interfere with.

The participants in the study exercised in two regimens. One group had two 20-minute sessions, four times a week while the other exercised for thirty to forty minutes in one session, also four times a week. Most of the participants were 55 or older, though, so younger people with insomnia can significantly increase the intensity of their exercise.

When it comes to aerobics and cardio, it's difficult to make your exercise too frequent. Just thirty minutes each day can do wonders, but if you can manage to do two such sessions every day of the week, perhaps once in the morning and once in the afternoon, your results could be much better and be felt sooner. Of course, if you are younger, it's also a good idea to go with the more intense alternatives to the exercises that the study used. Instead of walking, for example, young people can benefit from jogging.

Now, while increasing the frequency of your aerobic sessions is generally a good idea, you should beware that you don't make individual sessions too long and too intense. Running on a treadmill for too long can certainly upset your body and make it even more difficult to fall asleep. This is especially true if you're completely out of shape.

It's best to start small and take it one day at a

time while listening to what your body is telling you. You'll know best if you're pushing yourself too hard and if you need to cut back on your exercise. Furthermore, other forms of exercise and intense workouts such as weight lifting might not help alleviate insomnia, so you must remember to stay moderate. If you go about it in a gradual manner and stick to your routine, you can start seeing results anywhere between 4 and 24 weeks after you begin.

Apart from the popular wisdom, which postulates that getting tired through exercise promotes sleep, it's not exactly clear from a scientific perspective why exercise can alleviate insomnia. What we do know is that moderate aerobic exercise is especially beneficial if done later in the day. Some experts have suggested that the rapid rise in body temperature during exercise and the subsequent decline of it after the session might be the cause. At any rate, exercise is also known to be an excellent way to combat problems such as anxiety and depression, which, in turn, improves your sleep.

Yoga

At this point, virtually everyone has heard of Yoga, but a lot of people don't really know what it's all about. Since its beginnings in Northern India more than 5,000 years ago, this Hindu spiritual discipline has found its way to every corner of the developed world and deeply embedded itself into the popular culture. Yoga is much more than a popular cultural trend, though, as it has found its place in all manner of therapy, treatment, and physical exercise.

Yoga revolves around things like controlled breathing, basic meditation, and special physical postures. Yoga is about finding peace of mind, learning to relax, improving self –control and reliance, but it's also about fitness and flexibility. In the simplest terms, it has a range of benefits to mental and physical health alike.

As such, Yoga is also often applied in the treatment of insomnia because of its stress-reducing properties, among other things. The appeal of Yoga is also in that it's not a particularly intense exercise, so it's an excellent option if you want to try something that doesn't require you to exert yourself physically. It's not that you shouldn't exercise and do cardio, though, but Yoga can help you balance things out and not rely on aerobics and other workout routines as much.

The effects of Yoga on people with insomnia have been studied at Harvard Medical School. The participants that the researchers studied had problems of varying degrees and stemming from a range of different causes. The subjects were trained in basic Yoga routines and engaged in the exercise for eight weeks. For comparison, the researchers gathered an array of information about the issues that the participants were experiencing in the course of two weeks prior to the introduction of Yoga.

After the eight weeks had passed, the

researchers found that the quality of sleep for the participants improved significantly in more ways than one. Their sleep was more efficient and restful, for one, but they also slept longer and with fewer interruptions. On top of that, Yoga helped the participants fell asleep faster than before.

There were other studies that generally produced the same results. It also appears that Yoga, just like aerobic exercise, reduces sleepiness and drowsiness during the day. All of this is on top of all the other benefits that Yoga can introduce into your life. Depending on the practice, of which multiple exist, Yoga sessions can be a bit longer, often lasting for over an hour. The flip side is that it doesn't have to be practiced every day. Some of the studies made use of 75-minute sessions only twice a week, and the results were apparent. What's more, Yoga has been found to mend symptoms of insomnia among a wide range of groups, including older women, pregnant women, former cancer patients, younger adults, and many others.

What you can also do is change your personal regimen around and engage in shorter sessions just before bedtime each night. You can get started with some very simple poses at first to see how they affect you after a week or so. Keep in mind that Yoga can be a very broad term that encompasses a whole lot of different techniques, some of which are not meant to soothe but instead energize you.

All you need to get started are comfortable,

simple clothes and a thin exercise mat. The first pose you can try is called Viparita Karani, which is a very simple pose that requires you to stretch your legs up the wall while lying down. You will have to get close to the wall and keep your legs as straight as possible against the wall, essentially forming an L-shape with your body. You can hold this pose for around thirty seconds and focus on your breathing.

Another example is the lying butterfly pose. This pose also requires you to lie down on your back, but this time, you will do your best to put the bottoms of your feet together and let your knees go to the side, as close to the floor as possible. Keep your arms relaxed on the floor by your side and, as always, focus on your breathing. Another incredibly simple pose is lying down on your back, keeping your legs straight and flat, and your arms by your sides with palms facing upward. Focus on breathing deep and hold the pose a bit longer than thirty seconds since it's an easy one.

Combining these three poses into a quick bedtime routine is a tiny step, but it's definitely a starting point. To get the most out of Yoga, you will have to at least read a couple of tutorials or, ideally, join a group program or get a personal trainer. Yoga is incredibly popular and widespread, so it should be very easy to find more information or a program that works for you.

Staying on the Move

It's very important to move around. We weren't made to sit in cubicles, cars, and our armchairs at home for all our waking hours. Any longer walk is good for you, but certain environments are definitely better than others because they can boost the benefits you get from walking. Of course, the environments I'm talking about are those that are rich in nature. If you live near a forested area, then it's a no-brainer, but city parks can certainly be an effective substitute if nothing else is available.

Studies have shown that the time of day in which you take a walk can also affect the quality of your sleep. An afternoon or early evening walk is better than one in the morning. Ideally, your walk should end at least two or three hours before bedtime to give your body time to reduce its temperature and bring you down. Walking is exercise, after all, so most of the principles we mentioned earlier will apply.

When it comes to walking early in the morning, this exercise is certainly not without its benefits. A walk in the morning to make you more alert and lively and a walk in the evening to get you ready for bedtime is an excellent combination to combat insomnia from two sides. As for the walking sessions, 25 to 30 minutes should suffice as long as you don't walk too slowly. Another crucial aspect is regularity, so you should do your best to stick to a daily schedule as much as possible.

In general, walking will reduce your stress levels, alleviate symptoms of depression, and can also help exercise your back. Apart from improving the quality and ease of sleep, walks can also reduce daytime symptoms of insomnia such as drowsiness and give you more energy.

A great way to help you stick to a walking schedule and get the most out of your exercise is to get a pet dog. Not only will a pooch keep you up and around, but you will also be more likely to socialize with other people while walking. To that effect, Atlanta researchers at the Morehouse School of Medicine have conducted a rather large study on older adults who suffered from insomnia. They found that the incidence of insomnia was reduced by as much as 40% for those folks who socialized more and took walks.

Another excellent idea is to take your aerobic or Yoga exercise outdoors to a clean, quiet, natural environment. Not only will the environment be more relaxing than an apartment on a busy street, for instance, but you will also get cleaner air and more oxygen, which is always very important in exercise of any kind. Riding a bicycle through the woods or a city park is a great and quintessential approach to getting the most out of this time.

Overall, it will be very good for you to just take a thirty to sixty-minute timespan out of your afternoon and make it a special time that you spend on yourself, engaging in healthy activities. Don't take your work and your worries with you; leave these things at home and at the office.

If possible, you shouldn't take your phone along either since it will do little more than distract you and interrupt your relaxation time or, worse yet, your Yoga session. All of this isn't just about physical exercise. The unseen and equally important aspect of this routine will be the fact that you are taking care of yourself and taking steps to feel better. If you've been inactive and in terrible shape for a long time, then just starting to move around will feel like a great accomplishment. It will boost your morale and represent a reward in and of itself, but don't forget to keep at it and stick to the schedule.

Chapter Six: Digital & Visual Detox Steps

What we will discuss in this chapter is by far one of the most common bad habits that we have in contemporary society when it comes to our sleep routine. With the advent of television sets, this has been an issue for quite a while, but the emergence of smartphones and tablets has taken things to a whole new level.

Ask yourself how often you go to bed straight from your desktop PC or laptop, only to then whip out the phone and begin scrolling through social media or watching videos, sometimes with the TV on in the background as well. We are surrounded by screens from the moment we wake up to the moment our brains doze off. Most people think nothing of it, but studies have found that the light from these screens, particularly something called blue light, might severely impact your natural sleep cycle.

Digital Problems and Blue Light

Blue light, which is emitted by the digital devices we use in general, has been found to affect our levels of melatonin. This is a hormone that plays an important role in making your brain induce sleepiness. Using your smartphone and other similar devices throughout the evening and in bed might

64

reduce your ability to fall asleep but it's even more likely to hinder the quality of your sleep once you do manage to doze off. As such, the hours you spend looking at the touchscreen can make you wake up feeling tired and less alert. These issues have been presumed for a while, but the rise of the smartphone is a relatively recent phenomenon. The effects of blue light are still being studied and we are bound to find out even more about its effects on our biological mechanisms.

What's particularly tricky is that a lot of people tend to habitually use their smartphones or TVs to doze off. Indeed, scrolling through Internet pages on your phone or watching a TV show on a very low volume does seem to have certain sedative effects. Not only is this an evening ritual for many people, but polls have shown that some 60% of Americans like to watch television while falling asleep at least occasionally. One of the major electronics manufacturers, LG, actually conducted its own survey on this and found that 61% of those surveyed tend to fall asleep with the TV on.

The problem with your TV set, in particular, is mainly in the fact that it contributes to the aforementioned problem of your poor sleep hygiene. The main reason that a TV can make many people doze off is the background noise it provides when it's set on a lower volume. The noise that's set to a perfect volume can be just enough to drown out worries and recurring thoughts. Your TV can be even more soothing if you are watching something you've already seen many times because familiarity can be comforting.

So, what is the problem then? The problem goes back to blue light and its effect on your melatonin levels. Because of this, your sleep can be shallower and more fragile, keeping your brain semi-alert even when you're sleeping. This is how you end up spending less time in some very important stages of sleep or miss them altogether, leading to you feeling tired in the morning.

Besides, if you leave the TV on all night, something stimulating or louder can come on the program and wake you right up. If you do use your TV to rock yourself to sleep, you should definitely replace it with the infinitely better alternative that is music, like we discussed in the first chapter.

Another possible problem with television when it comes to insomnia is binge-watching. We live in a time of availability and abundance. It's so easy to get entire seasons of the most interesting shows in little more than an instant. As a study conducted by the University of Michigan showed, however, binge-watching your favorite show through the afternoon can leave your brain highly stimulated and unwilling to sleep. You should instead try to stick to the old ways as much as possible, which means watching one episode a day at most.

With all that being said, smartphones might be much worse than TVs. The connection between bedtime smartphone use and insomnia was studied at the University in California just a couple of years ago. The study found a significantly greater incidence of sleep latency among those participants who used their phone while in bed. The only problem with the findings is that some of these people might be using their phones because they couldn't fall asleep to begin with, not the other way around. Be that as it may, the effect of blue light on our melatonin levels was confirmed in numerous other studies.

The research is ongoing in this field, but the correlation has been all but established. As such, going screen-free for one to three hours leading up to bedtime is definitely something you should try. Digital devices like smartphones drive business and the economy as a whole has come to rely on the incredible level of connectivity that they provide between people, so they are here to stay. But, if you can do without them for a little while in the evening, the benefits to your sleep might be immense.

It's also worth pointing out that all light has the potential to mess with your melatonin levels, but blue light is significantly more troublesome than old fashioned light bulbs and such. Modern LED lights might be even worse. There is also ongoing research into the possibility of blue light increasing the risk of health problems other than insomnia as well, but we will probably have to wait a while for anything conclusive. One thing is for sure; the majority of people sleep best in darkness. If you are one of the people who require at least a dim light source while sleeping, you should keep that light to a minimum and try to gradually eliminate it.

Meditation as an Alternative

You have already learned about a number of things that can help you relax in the evening and doze off quicker, but there are many other strategies to cover. Instead of watching a movie or scrolling through social media pages, you should consider trying meditation.

The link between meditation, peace of mind, and improved sleep has been known for quite a long time. Meditation is now widely used for a whole range of emotional and mental problems, including insomnia. As such, there are many courses, online tutorials, apps, classes, groups, and personal trainers that can teach you anything from the simplest to some highly sophisticated forms of the practice.

Perhaps the best thing about meditation is that it's free of any potential side-effects or risks. With the right online resources, it can also be completely free to get into. Meditation is all about getting a firm grip on your mind and emotions while reducing stress and anxiety. In the simplest terms, the goal of meditation is usually self-mastery, as is evident by its long history in religious practices all over the world, particularly India and Asia. This means that meditation alone can be highly beneficial, but when it's combined with things like cognitive behavioral therapy for insomnia, the effects of the exercise can be even better.

How does meditation actually work, though? To keep it simple, meditation is about directing your mind toward a single focal point while pushing out everything else. This is why practitioners often "meditate on" a particular thing, be it an idol, a mantra, or their own breath. Using your breathing pattern as an object of focus in meditation is one of the simplest approaches.

The most important initial step is to be as comfortable as possible and rid your environment of most if not all distractions. All you need is some peace, quiet, and loose, comfortable clothing. You can use a mat on the floor and assume one of many positions. If you get into meditation, you will learn about a whole range of accepted poses that experts use, but you can start by simply sitting down on the ground with your legs crossed and your arms resting completely relaxed on your thighs or at your sides.

All you have to do then is to close your eyes, begin breathing slowly and deeply, and focus as intensely as you can on your breath. Pay attention to each time you inhale and exhale, but also try holding your breath in for a couple of seconds. Use your breath as something to fall back on if your mind starts to wander toward other thoughts, especially if they are your worries. You can try starting with a five to ten-minute session each night and see if it helps you relax after a few days.

Studies have found that meditation has the potential to exercise and bolster the areas of your brain that are in charge of sleep. Because of this, meditation won't just help you fall asleep faster but will also improve the depth and restfulness of your sleep. Of all the exercises and routines, meditation is one of the most effective ways of boosting your brain's melatonin production, but getting to that level might take some work.

Nonetheless, meditation could well be the ultimate solution for you, so it's definitely worth looking into. This is one of those things where you really have to persevere and prepare yourself for a slow onset of positive results. It might take you a lot of Internet browsing and reading or a whole bunch of trial and error, but the results that some folks have enjoyed certainly make it worthwhile.

Breathing Exercise

We already mentioned the most basic of breathing exercises a bit earlier, but this too is a field with a wide range of options and practices. Seeing as breathing exercises usually focus on alleviating stress, anxiety, or panic attacks, they can also yield results when you're trying to doze off.

A Harvard doctor by the name of Andrew Weil has proposed a very simple breathing exercise that he believes can put you under in as little as one minute. It's called the 4-7-8 breathing exercise and it basically boils down to breathing in a very specific way for sixty seconds. Breathing exercises as a means of fighting stress, insomnia, and anxiety are Dr. Weil's specialty, with a focus on the strong connection between breathing and the finer details of our physical and mental processes. Indeed, the way you breathe can make or break many aspects of your health and can even affect your mood.

The importance of proper breathing in this regard is what lies at the center of the 4-7-8 breathing exercise, also referred to as the "relaxing breath." Dr. Weil came up with this method while studying ancient meditative practices from India. The name of the technique comes from the length of each step of breath during the exercise.

The 4-7-8 technique has five steps and is incredibly simple and easy to do, but you'll need some general pointers first. For one, it's best to sit down and make sure that your back is straight because this will give your lungs the most room. Weil also advises that the practitioner puts the tip of their tongue just above the inner side of their upper teeth for the whole duration of the exercise. While you exhale, the air should go out around the sides of your tongue.

The first step is to exhale strongly, controllably, but fully, ideally making a subtle whooshing sound. After that, the next step is to close your mouth and inhale for a total of four seconds through your nose, as quietly as possible. You will then hold your breath for seven seconds. The fourth step is to exhale in the same way you did initially but over a period of eight seconds. The fifth step is to repeat the same breath four times. Make sure that you are focused solely on your breathing while doing this, and that's all there is to it.

The most decisive of these steps is the one where you will be holding your breath because this is when your body absorbs the oxygen that's processed in your lungs and attains the relaxing effect of the exercise. The simplicity of this exercise and the bold claims made by Weil as to its effectiveness sparked quite a bit of interest when he first came up with it. Other experts have since put this exercise to the test, and some of them certainly didn't fall asleep in sixty seconds. However, the very calming effect of Weil's breathing exercise has been noted across the board and the technique has been adopted by numerous sleep coaches and other therapists.

As usual, the technique will require practice and some trial and error before you can perfect it. Practice won't be a problem, however, seeing how simple and quick the exercise is. You should try doing it twice a day for a period of two months or so. The value of this exercise is both in its efficient utilization of oxygen and its meditative aspects, so it can be an effective way to combat stress in your daily life in general, not just your late evenings. At any rate, this is just one of the strategies that you can put together as part of your nightly routine, and it's certainly healthier than staring at a touchscreen.

Chapter Seven: Leading a Purposeful Life & Enjoying Contribution

In this chapter, we will move on to problems that are a bit more difficult to define and pinpoint but are common nonetheless. What I mean is that insomnia isn't always brought on by something particularly specific. There are many general, negative feelings that can torment us in our daily life, all of which can interfere with our sleep.

For instance, a general feeling of aimlessness and a lack of direction can weigh very heavily on many people's minds. Feeling stuck, empty, idle, and generally disoriented can get stressful or lead to depression, which is insomnia's greatest ally. When you feel better about yourself and your life, you will find it easier to relax and keep your mind at ease.

If you feel like your life is missing something and is devoid of meaning, purpose, and joy, then that might be your greatest problem. Sleep tends to be affected when you find it difficult to find a reason to even wake up in the morning, let alone feel fresh and upbeat.

More often than not, purpose won't just find you and put you on track, as this tends to work the

73

other way. You are the one who has to give your life a purpose. While that might seem like a gigantic undertaking, you should know that it starts with small steps and minor changes that you should introduce to your life. Still, acquiring a strong sense of purpose and direction will take time, as it might eventually lead to you having a whole new outlook on life.

Purposeful Days and Restful Nights

The studies that have been done in recent years have corroborated this link. Notably, the subject was studied at Northwestern University and Rush University Medical Center, Illinois.

Published in 2017, the study in question was conducted on older adults, but the researchers are confident that the results are likely to apply across the board, especially for adults. In the simplest terms, they found that having a purpose in life reduces the incidence of sleep disturbance and improves the overall quality of sleep in the long-term. According to the researchers, it's all about cultivating a purpose or a sense thereof, which they say can be grown and enhanced through things like mindfulness therapy.

The researchers focused on adults who were over sixty years of age because, as you know, the prevalence of insomnia among these folks is the highest. The study made use of 823 participants who were of sound mind and generally healthy. The participants were classified into those who reported a feeling of meaning and purpose in their lives and those who felt that purpose was lacking. They were also comprised of both men and women, and half the participants were African-American.

Of course, a feeling of purpose is a highly subjective matter, so the researchers came up with a 10-question survey that was given to all participants. The survey explored the subjects' feelings of fulfillment or lack thereof in relation to their past accomplishments and their outlook on the future. Each participant was also given a bigger questionnaire examining their sleep habits and quality. Those who reported having a purposeful life were found to be 63% less likely to have sleep apnea and the incidence of restless leg syndrome was also lesser. The quality of their sleep, in general, was also examined and found to be better than among those who felt their lives were meaningless.

One of the lead researchers thus concluded that a finding and cultivating a purpose in life is an effective way of combating insomnia without any drugs, particularly through mindfulness therapy. We'll get into this technique in more detail soon, but that's just part of the picture. The authors of the study also noted a correlation between a feeling of purpose and better health in general.

The state of your health can have major implications for your sleep pattern, so all of this is connected on some level. Anxiety and stress can have adverse effects on one's health, for example, and people who walk around with a purpose tend to

75

experience less of these two problems. And, of course, anxiety and stress also directly affect your ability to sleep.

Apart from helping you mentally, a purpose in life can also have physical effects on your lifestyle. Depending on what it is, a purpose can get you up and moving, going to great lengths and getting a lot of meaningful work done throughout the day. When we get a lot of things done during the day and we know why we did those things, not only do we get a sense of fulfillment but we also tend to be exhausted and naturally sleepy in the evening.

The following tips and information will help you reorient yourself and infuse your life with a sense of meaning. Still, there can be no clear and simple manual to help you find a purpose, as this is something that each individual has to identify personally. The tips we'll cover are generally changes that you can introduce into your life to help you increase your chances of finding a purpose, but you will have to know a purpose when you've found it.

It's not that it's particularly difficult to give your life meaning – it's that this journey is highly personal and will be unique to your experience. The important thing is to get started on a path, and the rest is bound to fall into place sooner or later. Perhaps the most important thing about having a purpose is that it gives you something concrete to think about, drawing your mind away from dreadful thoughts, stress, and anxiety. Leading an empty life and having too much time to think can be dangerous and it can certainly keep you up at night.

Finding Purpose in Life

If you happen to be someone who feels disoriented and lacking direction in life, you must be wondering how you can fix that and turn yourself around. As we mentioned, purpose and meaning can be cultivated at your own initiative. Just because you haven't "found yourself" by a certain age doesn't mean that there can be no purpose for you. As much as it might seem to be the opposite at times, life is indeed full of purpose on every corner – at least potential purpose.

What I mean is that purpose can come from surprising sources that you previously paid little attention to. We often obsess over concepts of higher purpose of some kind and set ourselves up for disappointment, but some folks manage to find meaning in little things. When life has you feeling directionless, the best thing to do is focus on the short term for a while and strive for three simple things: goals, schedules, and structure.

It's good to have a long-term goal in life, of course, but that's not necessary to get you started on a path. What you should do is choose one or multiple smaller goals that you can see yourself achieving in a relatively short span of time. Think about what you need in your life, such as changes that you would like to introduce. Do you need to get in shape? Do you want to write a novel? Do you wish to learn a new language? All of these are legitimate goals that can definitely make your days more fulfilled.

The second important aspect of your reorientation is schedule. Certainly, hectic and packed schedules nowadays are often a source of much stress and anxiety for many people, but that doesn't mean that having a schedule is a bad thing – quite the contrary. In fact, human beings generally thrive on schedules and they can help us get a lot more done in less time.

The feelings of aimlessness are much less likely to occur if your activities every day are a matter of schedule. You will know where you're going, what comes next, and what you need to work on. If you are trying to get in shape, for instance, you will have a great opportunity to make a schedule as this will require exercise, a well-planned diet, and other activities that go into a workout routine.

Don't limit yourself to just thinking about a few things that you'll do tomorrow. Your schedule should be written down for as long ahead as possible. You should try taking an entire week, writing down a number of activities and errands for each day. Make sure that your days are as filled up as possible and do your very best to stick to that schedule.

There are other things that can help you if you are finding it difficult to create a schedule. Pets are a great example, especially those that require certain activities such as dogs. A dog will give you something to look after and it will get you out on walks and all kinds of activities. Studies have shown that dog ownership has a wide range of benefits for physical and mental health. In fact, dogs have been used in therapy to help folks overcome depression and anxiety for quite a while now. Of course, you will have to take care that your pet doesn't interfere with your sleep at night.

In the end, schedules will give your life structure, which, in turn, will get you focused and oriented. Some folks might prefer to improvise and take things in life as they come, but human beings generally need to have a structure in their daily life. Sometimes, you have to force yourself into it and all of this can demand a major change in your habits and mentality, but it will be worth the effort. Waking up in the morning and knowing that your day is filled with activities will help you avoid the rabbit hole of negative thoughts. Simply put, you will be too busy to worry. By the time you're ready to go to bed in the evening, you will be able to reflect on a day that was productive and meaningful, and this is a very soothing feeling.

Trying out new activities is another great way to increase your chances of finding a purpose, even a special one. Instead of being inert and giving in to the false comfort of an unchanging life, you should strive to try as many new things as possible. The great thing about trying new activities is that you will be testing yourself and getting to know yourself better. New hobbies might well lead to an unexpected discovery of purpose and even a life's calling.

Of course, one of the greatest friends of purpose and meaning in human life is creation. Taking up a creative hobby is one of the best methods of filling up your leisure hours with meaningful activities. These hobbies can revolve around anything from various arts to things like carpentry and building. No matter how seemingly small or trivial they might seem, creative endeavors always have the potential to help you uncover talents you didn't know you had.

Generosity and Mindfulness

A sense of fulfillment and purpose is, of course, tied to overall happiness, and a source of happiness that's perpetually underrated is generosity. It's unfortunate, but generosity tends to take a backseat more and more often as the decades go by. For millennia, traditional wisdom has known that giving and helping others makes us happier and more whole, but this is something that has also been studied by experts in recent times.

Indeed, the positive effect that generosity has on our mental state might have been underestimated all along. In particular, we are talking about selfless acts, altruism, and helping others without expecting any reward. As a recent study conducted at the University of Zurich, Switzerland suggests, the reward is in the generous act itself or, rather, in the emotional effect it has on you.

As it turns out, a selfless act tends to activate certain areas of our brain, such as the ventral striatum, which is a part of your brain's reward system. This is why we feel satisfied and stimulated when we are generous even if we don't receive material compensation. In the study, this response was observed via an MRI scan but also the participants' reported subjective feelings.

The participants were divided into two groups, both of which were given a certain amount of money. One group was told to spend it all on themselves while the other was instructed to use it to help and give gifts to other people. The change in overall happiness was significantly more pronounced among the charitable group. As such, it would appear that conventional wisdom was right. Contributing to the wellbeing of others makes people feel fulfilled and is one of the greatest ways to acquire a sense of purpose. This is why charity and selflessness are a life calling for many folks.

Earlier, we mentioned that the study on purposefulness and sleeping disorders noted something called mindfulness therapy. In essence, mindfulness is a popular relaxation technique, somewhat meditative in nature. The goal is to make you more focused and present in the current moment, as opposed to worrying and stressing over other things. It's also an exercise that fosters awareness and concentration.

Mindfulness therapy generally makes use of

cognitive therapy, counseling, and various meditation techniques, including breathing exercises and other things, some of which we mentioned in the previous chapter. If this sounds like something you'd be interested in, there are many online courses and tutorials about mindfulness, but you can also look for personal trainers.

Overall, leading a purposeful life is all about making one's life more enjoyable and satisfying. Whatever the source of these feelings might be for you, enjoying a life with meaning and purpose is bound to reflect well on your ability to sleep. You shouldn't forget other small things that make life worth living, such as laughter. Laughing heartily and frequently can reduce the levels of cortisol in your brain and improve your emotional state in the long run.

Hi, I hope you're enjoying my book and you're starting to derive the benefits. Once again, I'd be very grateful if you could leave a review here ----------------

Thank you!

Tony

Chapter Eight: Avoid Afternoon Napping

Since insomnia often results from poor sleeping habits, it's going to be very important to tidy up these habits and pay more attention to your sleeping schedule. If your schedule is a mess or is non-existent, that's something that you're going to have to change drastically. That means you will have to improve upon your sleep hygiene quite a bit.

Afternoon naps, for instance, can be a pitfall that many folks fall into. When you already have insomnia, the chances are good that you're generally tired during daytime, which can make an afternoon nap seem like the logical, healthy thing to do, but this is often not the case. Such naps can make your sleep problems even worse and, seeing as it's often insomnia that brings you to that situation to begin with, this can be quite a vicious cycle.

As you can imagine, there is much more to sleep, naps included, than the average person knows. We'll go into more detail on the dos and don'ts of napping in this chapter, but we'll also take some time to help you learn more about your body's need for sleep and how all of that works exactly. In the process, you'll gain a better understanding of your body's sleep-related natural processes but also your insomnia.

The Intricacies of Sleep

The time you spend sleeping is a period when your body undergoes the necessary restoration. Your brain compartmentalizes and deals with a lot of the input that has accumulated during the day; it takes care of crucial processes in your body that remain unseen. So, while sleep is all about rest and rejuvenation, a lot of things are still going on under the surface.

We have learned much about sleep from the research that has been conducted over the decades, and sleep is now generally seen as a process that consists of two main phases, which are the rapid eye movement, or REM, stage and non-REM. People with a healthy sleep cycle tend to fall asleep within fifteen minutes after they hit the pillow and they go through the latter stage first.

The non-REM phase is usually divided into four stages ranging from the initial light sleep to deep sleep at stage four. This entire first phase, which usually lasts between 45 and 60 minutes, will slow your functions down, including brain activity, circulation, and heart rate. Your blood pressure will drop and your breathing will slow down. Your body might also experience involuntary movements, but that doesn't always happen.

Once you enter REM, your eyes will start to move around rapidly, as the name of the phase suggests. This occurs with your eyelids closed and the rest of your body in paralysis. While your breathing can slow down to a crawl during REM, your brain activity will spike, and this is the phase where you dream. To accommodate the heightened brain activity, your heart will be hard at work getting blood to it, which causes fluctuations in your heart rate and blood pressure.

Your REM phase will last roughly 30 to 45 minutes, at which point you will go back to non-REM. These phases will then proceed to alternate for the duration of your sleep. As you can see, both phases are important and carry with them crucial processes that get your body ready for the next day. Because of how complex your sleep is, quality is much more important than quantity.

Your sleep-wake cycle is a part of your 24-hour circadian rhythm or one side of it. If you've ever heard terms such as "internal clock" used colloquially, you should know that this is very much a real thing. Like other living beings, humans have their internal clock that regulates many processes that occur during the circadian cycle and corresponds to the cycle of night and day.

Indeed, there are many internal processes that occur around specific times of day in healthy people. Your body temperature and the levels of various hormones, for instance, fluctuate throughout the day and reach specific levels and particular times of day and night. As much as you might think that you're a night owl, there is no escaping the fact that the cycle of daylight and darkness determines our internal clocks. This is why traveling causes jet lag and people who live in or close to the Arctic Circle are especially prone to things like insomnia and depression.

Insomnia tends to occur when other factors interfere with the functioning of our circadian rhythm. As we discussed, medical conditions, anxiety, stress, and poor sleeping habits are some of the most common among these factors. Therefore, beating insomnia is all about getting yourself back in balance and readjusting your disrupted rhythm, which is why this change can sometimes take quite a while.

While insomnia is generally considered a sleep disorder, it can also be viewed as a symptom that often stems from larger problems. This is why a holistic approach and a change in many aspects of your lifestyle are required. You will have to identify the cause through trial and error and then address it with a long-term solution in mind. Just tackling the symptom with short-term answers will never get you back on track.

The Art and Dangers of Naps

All of this brings us to napping, which is one of the most common consequences of insomnia but also a frequent disruptor of our sleep-wake cycle. As pleasant and comfy as it might be, taking that afternoon nap can often be your worst decision of the day. Before we get into that, though, it's worth pointing out that naps aren't necessarily an evil that must be avoided at all costs, at least not by default. This is especially true for the elderly or folks who are sick.

Short "powernaps" can actually be quite useful and have little impact on your ability to fall asleep at night. These naps should be no longer than between 20 and 40 minutes and they should be had strictly within the time window between around 12 and 3 PM. Even so, you shouldn't get these quick naps unless you're absolutely positive that it's necessary. And if your insomnia is severe, it's best to avoid naps altogether.

If you do manage to get it right, though, this quick powernap in the early afternoon can give you the boost you need to get through the day with more alertness and energy. You might even catch up on a few things that you've missed last night, but don't forget that taking powernaps in the early afternoon is no substitute for a good night's rest. As such, if these naps become habitual, you might have a problem.

When doing an early powernap, the important thing is not to let it get out of hand and turn into a sleeping session that started as a mere powernap. If you're an insomniac who isn't getting quality sleep, the urge to pass out in the afternoon can sometimes be quite strong.

Don't be fooled, though, as this is no way to make up for your restless nights and will only make things worse in the long run. Not only will your sleep quality be poor the following night just like before but you might not get any sleep at all. Even though it's probably your disrupted circadian rhythm that is making you crave a nap in the afternoon, giving it what it wants will only push you further down the rabbit hole.

It's also worth noting that afternoon sleepiness often occurs naturally with people who don't necessarily suffer from insomnia. Essentially, the processes of your circadian rhythm that regulate your sleepiness and keep you going through the day can often slow down for a while in the earlier afternoon, making you drowsy. This effect should wear off not too long after the initial onset of sleepiness, so it might be best to ignore it and wait for your rhythm to rev up again.

Not only is the rhythm bound to slow down again later in the evening, but the sleepiness is likely to be stronger if you take no naps. Furthermore, if the onset of drowsiness really is caused by the natural slowdown of your circadian rhythm, the subsequent uptick will come whether you take a powernap or not. The problem is that, with insomnia, you never know what the real cause is, so the safest bet is perhaps to avoid indulging any nap requests from your brain.

The question thus seems to be whether or not you should take naps at all, even if they are short and well-controlled. Simply put, if you already suffer from insomnia and are a younger adult, you should probably refrain from naps altogether. The strongest emphasis, however, is on avoiding afternoon naps. Overall, if you have trouble sleeping at night, daytime naps are one of the first things you should eliminate.

Apart from young children, the elderly and the ill are the only groups of people who truly need naps, with the possible addition of pregnant women. If you happen to be pregnant, you shouldn't worry yourself too much about a few restless nights or catching some Z-s in the afternoon, especially if you have no history of insomnia or other sleep disorders prior to the pregnancy.

It's important for pregnant women to be rested, of course, but your doctor and your body will know best if you need to introduce certain changes. Pregnant women are something of a unique case when it comes to most of these strategies in general. The cause of their insomnia is rather apparent and unlikely to last more than a few months, so it's not really something to be alarmed by.

Additional Tips

The difficulty in resisting the urge to doze off is often in the fact that we find ourselves sedentary in those situations. If it's 7 PM and you are at home after work, sitting in your armchair covered with a blanket, and you feel a sharp rise in sleepiness, it can seem impossible to resist.

As difficult as it might sound, the best thing you can do in that situation is to get up and moving. Instead of dozing off and ruining your chances of a restful night, you should go outside and take a walk, for example, ideally in a natural environment as we discussed earlier. This has to be a swift and strong decision on your part, and the problem is that it's often very easy to find excuses not to do it.

Sometimes it's cold outside, at other times it's too hot, but excuses are always abundant for the unwilling. Besides, if the conditions outside are truly hostile to human life, a walk isn't the only physical activity you can engage in to fight off the onslaught of sleepiness, as you well know. You might also be inclined to turn back to your old habits and use stimulants such as caffeine to keep yourself going through the afternoon, but it's not worth it.

Not only will caffeine do little to bring down an overwhelming sleepiness attack but it will also linger in your system for hours, as we discussed earlier. You will gain very little and just end up risking another night of light and interrupted sleep that leaves you tired in the morning.

Furthermore, late afternoons are not the only instance when you should never take a nap. Napping in the early morning, not long after you've woken up, is another bad idea, especially if you've slept for the average required seven to nine hours.

If you do opt for that quick powernap, remember what we said about the phases of sleep. The non-REM phase might last a while, but it goes from light to deep sleep, and you don't want to reach the latter. While a powernap could work at up to 40 minutes long, the ideal is 15 to 20. You should also add to that another 10 to 15 for getting back up to speed after waking up, particularly if you are doing work.

It goes without saying that waking up from a quick nap can leave you rather crusty and unfocused, so it's always a bad idea to nap just before doing something that requires attention and concentration. Being sleep deprived can often be better, safer, and more productive than post-nap drowsiness, which goes double for driving vehicles or operating machinery.

You will also want to avoid naps at all costs upon landing after a long flight, especially if it's in the afternoon. As mentioned earlier, traveling and jet lag have quite an impact on your circadian rhythm and it will need time to recover – time which will be prolonged if you go for a nap the moment you arrive in your hotel room.

The biggest lesson to take away from naps is that a recurring and powerful daytime need for them is a strong indicator that there's something wrong with your sleep. Giving in to the desire means you will essentially be feeding and cherishing the problem instead of addressing it. Despite the modest number of benefits that powernaps can provide, as an insomniac, you should consider them the very last resort as they aren't much better than sleeping pills when it comes to fixing your issue in the long-term. As you have seen by now, there are numerous alternatives that will actually help you toward beating your insomnia as well as get through the day.

Chapter Nine: Avoid Eating and Drinking in the Evening – Enjoy Highly Nutritional Foods during the Day

In addition to exercise and sleep, your diet is the third piece of the puzzle of healthy living. As usual, a healthy diet is another thing that modern living makes difficult for many people. We skip meals, we have back-to-back meals, we eat on the fly, and we often fail to give our body the amount of nutrition it needs. Minding what and how much you eat is important, but it also matters *when* you eat.

Eating late in the evening or just before you go to sleep has been known to cause issues for quite a while now, especially if we're talking about a full, strong meal. Your body has much less work to do when there's no food to digest, so it stands to reason that you should avoid a hefty meal before bed if you're having trouble falling asleep.

What food can do is upset your stomach, wake you up for the bathroom, stimulate your brain, and do a bunch of other things that interfere with sleep. Some foods are much worse in this regard than others, though, and we'll take a look at some of them soon. Overall, eating just before bed is not recommended even for the strongest of sleepers, let alone insomniacs. Of course, that doesn't mean that you should go to bed starving, but your dinner should be timed so that you give your body at least a few hours to process everything you've eating before dozing off.

Another set of problems with food are allergies, which don't always cause a rash, asphyxiation, or nausea. Allergic reactions can sometimes lean toward the subtle side, and these can be hard to detect on your own. Something you're eating might be having a particularly troublesome effect that's unique to you without you even realizing it.

An allergy is one of those medical issues that can and should be confirmed or ruled out with a doctor during the initial consultation about your insomnia. A doctor will probably inquire about your diet and try to see if you're allergic to anything, but if they don't, you should certainly ask about the possibility.

Foods to Avoid

There are certain foods that are known to hinder our ability to fall asleep, and this effect that they have is largely universal for all people. Some of them might surprise you and some are likely to be your favorites, but the good news is that you don't have to remove them entirely from your diet. In fact, what's particularly surprising is that some of these foods are otherwise healthy, so you wouldn't want to eliminate them anyway. The important thing is to just avoid them for a few hours leading up to bedtime.

Tomatoes, the quintessential vegetable and the main ingredient in many a salad, are one problematic food for your sleep. Certain amino acids that are found in tomatoes, such as tyramine, will prompt your brain to release chemicals that stimulate it and boost its activity. As surprising as that might be, the tomato is thus something of a stimulant, just like soy sauce, eggplants, red wine, and certain old cheeses, all of which contain the same amino acid.

Speaking of acid, many obviously acidic fruits are to be avoided before sleep as well, such as grapefruit, which has been known to sometimes cause heartburn if eaten before bedtime. Many fruits and vegetables with a high content of water should also be avoided so as to reduce your chances of waking up due to nature's call. Celery, cucumbers, and watermelons, with the last being quite a no-brainer, are some examples.

Beware the foods that are hard to stomach, meaning highly fatty or fried foods. French-fries, deep-fried foods, bacon, and anything else you can think of along those lines should be avoided at all costs. Of course, even worse are meals that incorporate two or more such ingredients, meaning pizza, eggs and bacon, and other heavy meals.

As you may or may not know, dark chocolate usually contains caffeine, so it is a bad idea to eat it before bedtime, especially in large quantities. A moderate, daily intake of dark chocolate is actually good for you, but there's no need to reduce your chances of falling asleep at night by munching on it in the evening.

Candy, in general, is problematic because it contains a whole lot of sugar that can upset your body. When you eat things like gummy bears or other candy, the levels of sugar in your blood will soar quickly and then fall back down fast once your insulin rises to meet the sugary challenge. These fluctuations can have a dramatic effect and prevent you from falling asleep or wake you up after you doze off.

You should also beware of the fact that caffeine can be found in many foods and drinks where you wouldn't expect it. Carbonated soft drinks such as coke and quite a few other sodas actually have caffeine in them, plus they can get your bladder going, none of which is good when it comes bedtime. Of course, you should never go to bed dehydrated, but if you want a tasty beverage at a later hour, you should always check the label, where caffeine contents will be noted.

Broccoli is another foodstuff you should avoid before bedtime. Its high content of fibers and sugars, some of which are indigestible, can easily cause sleeping problems. Broccoli is healthy and highly nutritious, of course, but it's best to stick to it during the day. Cauliflower and other similar vegetables are largely the same in this regard.

These are only some of the foods that can be particularly troublesome, but there are many others. If you've just found that you do eat some of them late at night, then you should stop doing that immediately. Since it's impossible to list every problematic food right now, your best bet is to just keep in mind what we said about late-night eating in general. If your dinner is not particularly heavy, it shouldn't take more than three hours for your body to stop working intensely on digesting the meal. At that point, you'll have a much easier time falling asleep.

Foods That Might Help

With all that being said, it can still sometimes be good to have a quick and small snack before bed, but only if that snack consists of some very special foods. There are also some things that are good to drink in the evening, as they can help induce sleep the natural way. If you're already the kind of person who doesn't eat before bed, maybe you will want to give some of these foods a try. It'll also be a good idea to add them to your dinner as an extra or just use them to replace some of the things you eat.

First and foremost, certain herbal teas can be quite good at inducing sleepiness in some people. They won't knock you out or anything, but they just might relax you and alleviate some of your anxieties enough for you to drift away. Chamomile tea, for instance, is a popular and widely accessible option. If you've never had it before, you'll be glad to know that its flavor is pleasant and   that it's very healthy.

One of the first cited benefits of chamomile tea is that it contains certain antioxidants that can suppress and help prevent inflammations. Furthermore, this tea can give your immune system a boost and alleviate symptoms of anxiety and depression, the two big enemies of sleep.

Apigenin is one of chamomile's antioxidants that can help induce sleepiness and combat insomnia. Studies have found that two doses of 270 milligrams a day can help adults fall asleep faster and be less likely to wake up during the night. Multiple studies have been done on this, and correlations were found among men and women alike. Another herbal tea worth trying comes from passionflower. It contains similar antioxidants and has been found to alleviate anxiety as well.

Foods that are high in protein are generally not recommended late at night, as we discussed, but there might be exceptions. Turkey meat is one potential candidate, though its role in inducing sleepiness hasn't been studied in experiments that deal with sleep specifically. However, turkey has tryptophan, which is an amino acid that makes your brain produce more melatonin, your sleep-inducing hormone. If you tend to get hungry before bed, you can try having a bit of turkey, but you shouldn't eat too much. And if you notice that it's not helping, it's best to put it back on the list of things that you don't eat before bed.

Also highly nutritious as well as very healthy,

almonds are another food that you should try introducing. Almonds are a source of antioxidants, fiber, fats, and many other things that make it a very wholesome source of nutrition. Almonds will also make your brain produce more melatonin to help you sleep. A very important aspect of almonds is that they contain a lot of magnesium, which has a whole range of benefits, including the potential to improve your sleep. This is because magnesium, like the teas we mentioned, can reduce inflammation as well as stress hormones. As always, you shouldn't overdo it, as one handful or about one ounce should be enough in the evening.

There is a range of other foods and drinks that you can try in moderation to see if they help, such as kiwi, tart cherry juice, walnuts, white rice, salmon, tuna, and much else. If you do believe that your case of insomnia might be helped with a dietary change, you can certainly experiment with some or all of the foodstuffs we just covered. The important thing to remember is to stay moderate and not give your body too much to work with at night, no matter how good the food might be for inducing sleepiness.

Other Dietary Advice

First and foremost, the best way to avoid the wrong foods and ensure that you eat sleep-friendly ones is to know exactly what to look for. Since we can't go over every single food or drink in this chapter, we'll take a look at those subtle ingredients that nature puts in there, which make some foods a better choice than others.

Keeping a healthy diet and minimizing your diet's negative effects on your ability to sleep is all about those hormones, enzymes, nutrients, chemicals, and amino acids. The things to look for are tryptophan, melatonin, gamma-aminobutyric acid (GABA), magnesium, potassium, calcium, pyridoxine, serotonin, histamine, folate, zinc, copper, antioxidants, acetylcholine, and, of course, certain vitamins such as D and B.

These are the factors that determine how a certain food affects you, but don't worry: you don't have to be a chemist, biologist, or nutritionist. Keep an eye on the labels of the things you buy and, if you're unsure about a certain food that interests you, scour the Internet for other people's input. Remember that there are millions of other people who struggle with the same issues, and they all have valuable experience to share.

In general, it's important to point out that your diet as a whole can have a dramatic effect on your sleep. We just covered numerous foods that you should avoid before bedtime, but you must understand that just ceasing to eat this stuff late at night might not be enough to solve your problem. You can't just eliminate candy from your nightly routine but continue eating the worst possible foods throughout the day while expecting things to change.

Since almost half of Americans report at least an occasional case of insomnia, the question is how much of that can be connected to their diet. Just like insomnia, unhealthy diets are a major problem that affects society in general. Many of our processed foods contain a high level of fat and salt while providing little nutrition. Especially problematic are sugars and their omnipresence in the things we eat and drink. Our reliance on sugar is incredibly dangerous and is known to cause a whole set of problems other than insomnia, some of which can be life-threatening.

You certainly have to maintain a nutritious diet through your days to keep you going, but instead of relying on a quick snack that makes your blood sugar go crazy, you should look to healthier, natural alternatives. Another good idea is to spread out your food intake for a more balanced diet. The traditional 3-5 meals per day are not always ideal. Our meals are often too big with long gaps in between. This shocks the body and keeps the nutrients in your body going up and down all the time. You should try to eat less but more frequently to keep yourself satiated and balanced throughout the day. It's also important to stay hydrated during the day, so make sure that you drink enough water, but don't overdo it before sleep for obvious reasons.

If you're aiming for a healthy diet that revolves around meat and veggies, then make sure that you avoid fatty meats like pork. You should stick with lean meat such as chicken. In general, the only fatty meat that doesn't have the potential to meddle with your sleep is fish, as we discussed earlier. Try to get your proteins and your carbs as naturally as possible.

Of course, pregnant women should take extra care when experimenting with their diet. If that happens to be your situation, you can certainly use all the advice that we have covered thus far, but you should always consult with your doctor before making changes in your diet. Overall, dietary changes, even when they are for the better, can be a shock for anyone's body, so it's always good to take your time and experiment one day at a time. When it comes to removing outright harmful substances from your life, however, the sooner you do it the better.

Chapter Ten: An Evening Orgasm Greatly Assists Restful Sleep

Whether you've heard about it before or not, this strategy is another one of those that have been around in popular wisdom for quite a while. Nowadays, though, there's also plenty of science to back up the claim that orgasms definitely promote sleep in our brains. Having an orgasm before bedtime can make you fall asleep faster and stay sleeping through the night. That goes both for sex and masturbation, although the effects on your brain and body aren't always identical between the two.

Orgasms are good for your health beyond just helping you overcome insomnia, though, but their effect on your sleep is particularly noteworthy. In fact, the quality of your sleep and your sex life tend to feed into each other quite a bit, both positively and negatively, depending on the circumstances. While an orgasm improves your sleep, restful nights will help you maintain a healthy sex drive. And so, in the event that one of these important aspects of your life is a struggle, it's a good idea to try and focus on fixing things in the other department.

One of the ways in which an orgasm helps you fall asleep is similar to many of the other strategies we covered. An orgasm will clear your head and usually give an instant relief of stress because it will make it difficult for you to think about other things. Even though it might stave off troubling thoughts only for a short while, that time might be just enough for you to doze off.

Sleep and Sex Life

There are two main ways in which insomnia can affect our sex lives. First and foremost, when your body and brain are deprived of sleep, your brain reduces its production levels of estrogen, testosterone, and other sex hormones, while ramping up cortisol, which, as you know, is a stress hormone. It doesn't take a neuroscientist to see how this imbalance can decimate one's sex drive.

On the other hand, insomnia's companion problems such as anxiety and depression will often not only suppress your sex drive but can also lead to sexual dysfunction on both the physical and mental plains. These mental disorders and hormone imbalances love to make each other worse, and they can both lead to some serious problems on the physical side of sexual dysfunction. Erectile dysfunction and even infertility are only some of the issues that can arise. Furthermore, the connection between sex life and sleep can be even more pronounced in women. This is because, with women, there are additional factors that can complicate things, such as pregnancy and menopause.

On the flip side, a dysfunctional or non-existent sex life can be a source of significant turmoil and dread for many people. If combined with a lack of social life in general, this lack of human contact and intimacy can weigh heavily on one's mind and lead to depression. Masturbation can be a very healthy outlet in such situations, but that too has its potential drawbacks.

Namely, masturbation is healthy in essence, especially for men, but it can be overdone, become a habit, and lead right back to depression. This is especially true when Internet pornography is involved in the mix. In recent years, there has been a significant surge in research and advocacy when it comes to the effects that Internet pornography can have on one's brain. The abundance and ease of access to this form of instant gratification are proving to be highly addictive for many. In many cases, psychological addiction can be much more insidious and difficult to deal with than physical dependence.

A dependence on this content to achieve gratification and relief can be rather dangerous, especially for men. There is a growing body of evidence that suggests that porn addiction also leads to depression and sexual dysfunction. In severe cases, insomnia will be the least of the problems. So, if you end up relying on masturbation, you should do your best to keep it moderate and as natural as possible. As a general rule of thumb, anything up to five times a week is healthy, and you should ideally use no visual stimulation or at least keep it mild and basic.

At any rate, masturbation should serve as a great way to bridge the gap and keep reaping the benefits of sexual release while you're in the process of finding a partner. Needless to say, sexual release is just one of the benefits of having intimacy in your life. There are all kinds of interactions in relationships that promote the production of feel-good hormones, ease the mind, reduce stress, and just improve your outlook on life in general.

Having someone to talk to about your problems, happy moments, hopes, dreams, and other things that are important to you will bring light into anybody's life. Spending time together while going for a walk or cuddling and all those other small things that make a relationship are all but necessities for a fulfilled human life. This remains one of the best safeguards against stress and depression, and it's a surefire way of improving your sleep as well.

Your Brain on Orgasm

The positive effects that an orgasm will have on your sleep and your brain in general mostly have to do with the hormones involved in the process. When you experience an orgasm, your brain will ramp up the production of a range of hormones that are related to feelings of calm, sleepiness, relaxation, reward, and much else. It's essentially a cocktail bomb of all that feel-good stuff that our brain can produce to put us at ease.

One of the more famous of these hormones is

oxytocin, which is colloquially known as the love hormone. This hormone is produced in various contexts, such as when we're spending quality time with our partner, or when a mother is interacting with her child. This pleasant and calming hormone may well have sedating effects that could be the main reason why an orgasm induces sleepiness since the orgasm significantly increases the hormone's secretion in the brain.

It seems that this hormone plays a crucial role in human bonding, and it also suppresses the production of cortisol, keeping stress to a minimum. Another orgasm-induced hormone is vasopressin, which also reduces your levels of cortisol even further. On top of that, vasopressin also reduces feelings of pain, which is why an orgasm can help alleviate problems like migraines and a bunch of other issues that could be keeping you up at night. It doesn't have to be a migraine either. A plain old headache or stomachache could be swept away or at least alleviated via an orgasm.

Serotonin, the quintessential feel-good hormone, is a neurotransmitter that's also plentiful during orgasm. Serotonin is a chemical that plays a very important role in your sleep cycle, particularly in the deep stage of your non-REM phase. Furthermore, a lack of serotonin is a dangerous chemical imbalance that is a common cause of clinical depression. As such, anything that brings up serotonin is very healthy for your mind and body.

While serotonin helps during non-REM, a hormone by the name of noradrenaline works to improve the efficiency and quality of the REM phase. When both of these hormones are secreted in appropriate quantities and balanced well, your sleep's quality will be optimal. Orgasms also tend to increase the levels of estrogen in women, which is another hormone that facilitates REM.

Then there are the hormones linked to sexual satisfaction such as prolactin. On the female side of things, prolactin also affects the intensity of the orgasm. Its more pertinent property, however, is sedation. This has been tested on lab rats in experiments where the test animals were injected with prolactin only to get drowsy and sometimes doze off. With that said, prolactin serves primarily to increase the production of milk after a woman gives birth, but the brains of both men and women who aren't pregnant will produce this chemical. There's also the after-sex hormone called nitric oxide, which is physically relaxing especially for men.

Orgasm has the potential to change your whole emotional state, give a sudden sense of clarity, and turn your mind around by 180 degrees. Researchers in the Netherlands have made some very interesting findings that pertain to female orgasm. It would seem that, during orgasm, most women were essentially cut off from experiencing emotions. The part of the brain where things like anxiety and fear originate is basically shut down during the orgasm. This isn't a long period of time, of course, but the switch that occurs during orgasm can seemingly change a woman's emotional state and sweep away any worries.

Other Benefits and Tips

As briefly mentioned earlier, orgasms and sex, in general, have a range of positive effects for your health as a whole. While it can hardly compare to an actual exercise regimen, sex itself can be viewed as a form of cardio. Apart from the physical activity involved, an orgasm will get your heart pumping, your blood pressure surging, and your breathing rate increasing, all of which are the makings of a cardio exercise. Orgasms are also excellent for your circulation in general.

For women, the complex nature of their sexuality can make the orgasm a very important concept in life. This is especially true for women who find it difficult to experience an orgasm. Learning how to have that experience can thus be an exercise in self-discovery and provide a feeling of achievement on top of everything else. In fact, some experts have argued that this can improve a woman's confidence and boost her emotional intelligence. This pertains especially to orgasms achieved through masturbation and, as such, can also foster a woman's sense of independence.

As you can probably gather, orgasms are unlikely to cure a severe case of insomnia in the long term. However, the sedating, sleep-inducing effects are doubtless. As such, an orgasm might be one of the best sleeping pills that nature has to offer. The effect is immediate, the side-effects are virtually non-existent, and there's hardly anything to get addicted to. Furthermore, it's impossible for your ability to fall asleep to become dependent on orgasms and, most importantly, there's no chance of having a terrible insomnia rebound that can happen after a while of relying on sleeping pills.

For all men and a great number of women, introducing an orgasm into the evening routine is also a very easy change to implement. It costs nothing, is completely natural, and is essentially foolproof. Having a significant other is definitely the superior option, but most of the benefits we just covered can be attained through masturbation at least to some degree, so there's hardly anything stopping you.

For the guys reading this, it's also worth reiterating the dangers of that fairly rare situation where the relationship between orgasms and sleep can be negative. The one thing you should not do is try and use masturbation as an outlet for greater problems or a means of filling a larger void in your life. Despite the sedating properties that an orgasm has, you should look elsewhere for fulfillment in life.

Don't engage in masturbation because you're bored and don't turn it into a chronic self-medicating activity. For that, you should look toward the many other strategies that we have covered, such as exercise, creative endeavors, meditation, yoga, and a million other productive activities that can get you up and running.

While it's easier said than done, improving your sex life is ultimately another great strategy to improve the quality of your sleep. If you're single, there isn't much advice that can be given other than to keep searching for that special someone and persevere through disappointments. Such is dating life, and we all have to get used to it.

However, there are many folks out there who are in relationships or are married, sometimes for a long time, yet they still aren't satisfied with their sex lives. If you can relate to that, then you know where you should focus. Since you are now aware of the strong bond between sleep and sex life, this will be something that you can take up with your partner or spouse. Don't shy away from having this conversation with them and letting them know that you have reason to believe that the lackluster sexual relationship is a source of physical discomfort for you. Relationships have to be refreshed sometimes, and it might be just the thing that both of you need.

Chapter Eleven: Seek Help if Your Relationship Is Causing You Stress

Apart from work, our relationships tend to be the other most important aspect of our lives. They are something we build throughout our lives and dedicate enormous amounts of energy to. As such, their stress potential is also incredibly high, and troubled relationships are generally a major contributor to sleep disorders among people from all walks of life.

Just like anxiety or stress in general, a dysfunctional relationship is one of those things that can work in unison with insomnia to create a vicious cycle, as they feed into each other perfectly. A troubled relationship can make it difficult for you to sleep, your inability to sleep can make you irritable and unstable, and so the cycle goes around, making itself worse every day.

If an important relationship in your life is going awry and is the cause of your sleepless nights, that's a problem you will have to resolve before you can get a good night's rest. Of course, this also happens to be one of the hardest steps in this book, but there's a way out of anything.

Fixing some relationships can take years, but you should not despair. Even if a relationship is dysfunctional, there are ways of altering your perspective and dealing with the stress that this problem causes. This means taking measures to reduce the effect that this negativity is having on you or, in other words, preliminary damage control in your self-interest. Finally, it's often a very good idea to seek help from a third party when things get really bad.

Reduce the Effect of Negativity

And so, the first important step is to do your best not to let dysfunctional relationships affect you too much. Of course, that doesn't mean shutting the person out or acting like the problem doesn't exist, which is the worst thing you could possibly do. It just means not letting it affect you in a way that grinds your life to a halt and ravages you with stress to the point where you can't function during daytime, let alone at night when you're locked in with your thoughts.

The perspective with which you look upon these problems can make a world of difference in how affected your life ends up being. It might seem counter-intuitive, but whenever you are trying to fix a broken relationship, you should start by asking yourself some simple yet important questions. For one, try and take an objective look at whether the problem is with you or the other person, but do so while not thinking about how they made you feel or any other emotional aspect of the issue. Make no mistake, though, this isn't to say that you should start by blaming yourself, quite the contrary. It's just that when it comes to the people we love, emotions can be

113

absolutely blinding and even the most rational man or woman can find themselves in delusion.

This is all in the interest of identifying the exact problem in the relationship. Understanding the full nature of the problem will quickly get your brain started working toward potential solutions and it will make you feel less lost and hopeless. There's hardly anything as stressful and devastating as seeing an incredibly important relationship begin to crumble and not even knowing what is going on or why it's happening.

Once you identify the problem and if you manage to place it in the other end of the relationship, you can begin doing your best to look at objective reality. You will likely become less shook, less obsessive, and much more rational. If you are consumed by anger, a thirst for vengeance, or judgment, you will have to cool down.

The best way to do this is to think of your significant other as that which they are – a human being. Human beings are imperfect and prone to losing their way, but they are also often blinded by emotions or complexes. You shouldn't give in to feelings of victimhood, as appealing as that might be.

Instead, you should change your perspective to one that is more compassionate both for you and your significant other. Always ask yourself if you are overreacting and keep your rationality in under scrutiny. High emotions can be an aggravating factor or even the cause of relationship problems, and they are impossible to suppress, but it's paramount to do your best to remain rational.

Of course, relationships can also be harmed by external factors that really aren't anybody's fault. In these situations, it's much easier to identify the problem and work together toward overcoming that hurdle. Whatever the situation might be, you should try and humanize both yourself and your loved one as much as possible. This will significantly reduce your stress levels and make the situation feel much more manageable.

Once you feel that you have a better mental grip on the situation and a deeper understanding of all the parts of the equation, you can start working actively toward reducing your daytime stress through the numerous strategies we have covered thus far.

The key is to stay functional and not allow other parts of your life to suffer and degrade. The more you let stress consume you and the more your life begins to destabilize beyond just the troubled relationship, the more you'll feel like you are losing all control. Besides, when you're consumed by stress and anxiety, the loss of control can be more than just a feeling. You might start making mistakes in numerous areas of your life and running many things in the process. Of course, all of this will exponentially increase your instability and sense of hopelessness. The nightly tossing and turning will thus get even worse, and life can assume a whole new shade of terrifying when you're chronically sleep-deprived.

Don't forget that insomnia makes you irritable and can impair your judgment while prolonged sleep deprivation can make you outright irrational. This is why it's important to question yourself objectively. It's entirely possible that the problems in your relationship began with an insomnia-influenced change in behavior on your part.

Your insomnia, in turn, could have been caused by some of the many other causes we have covered. That's why it's so important to do your best to work on improving your sleep while also looking to mend the problems in your relationship. You are now equipped with many strategies to combat stress whatever its cause might be, so you should use them. Once you start getting some rest and feeling better, you might realize that your problems aren't as bad as they seemed – you never know.

Reviving the Bonds

Once you have adopted the right mindset, identified the problem, and prepared yourself to deal with the issue, you can focus on actually trying to fix the relationship. The only question, of course, is how you are supposed to go about it.

What Tolstoy once wrote about families, in general, is also very true about relationships: all the happy ones are alike and each unhappy one is unhappy in its own unique way. There is a lot of conventional wisdom and many rules that apply across the board and can be used by all, but your personal relationship problems will require your own personal touch and specific approach. There's a whole lot that goes into fixing a failing relationship, no matter if it's with a partner, a parent, a child, or any other loved one.

The first thing to note, which I can hardly overstate, is the importance of communication. Of course, that might have occurred to you already as relationships are a form of communication in their own right. However, the breakdown of communication is perhaps the most common cause of relationships falling apart. And so, you need to ask yourself if you have really communicated with your significant other in a meaningful way and, if so, what was it that brought you two to this situation?

If you can't answer this question quickly and clearly, then the communication has failed between you and the other side, assuming that you both do agree that there is a problem. If your relationship is causing you stress and you're still unsure why, then you need to tell that to the other person so you can try to get to the bottom of it together.

Something that many people unfortunately don't understand is that communication is just as much about listening as it is about talking. You need to pay close attention to what your significant other or family member is telling you and vice versa. If the other person is dismissive or inattentive – tell them. If they like to interrupt you and always talk over you –

tell them. You should simply talk about every single thing that's bothering you. Assuming that this is a relationship that both sides value despite disagreements, your loved one will start paying attention if you're insistent. You must also make sure that you aren't the one who's being difficult.

You should also remember to make your perspective as positive as you can. Don't always focus on the negatives if you don't have to. A strong and prolonged focus on negativity can make you miss all that's good in life and magnify the problems in your perception. You should try and laugh with your loved one as often as possible and think about all the good times that you've shared. It's also a good idea to try doing an activity that you have never done before. Sometimes, we just need some time to bond again when life drives a wedge in between.

When discussing or arguing about your problems, you should avoid bringing up the past. For one, doing this rarely serves any purpose other than to attack, hurt, and insult. Secondly, if that particular thing from the past bothered you that much, you wouldn't be there in the relationship today, so it comes across as hypocritical and just needlessly escalates the conflict.

You should always strive to deescalate every conflict that you can. When it comes to spouses, family members, or the closest of friends, there is a powerful bond there, and the mere reminder that this bond exists can help calm things down. Try to remind both of you of all the experiences you've shared and all the intimate things you know about each other. These things have an incredible value that can't be dismissed even in the heat of an argument.

One thing you should remember is that heated arguments and passion, even if it's spiteful or otherwise negative at times, is a sign of that strong bond. The opposite of love is not anger or even hatred, but indifference. When two people who used to be close can sit in silent contempt and with no interest in discussing any of the issues, then the problem is much greater than when they argue.

While there's little you can do with true indifference, passion can always be converted and channeled into something good and loving, no matter how much negativity is in the air at a given moment. You just have to remind yourself of why you both care so much, even if the realization comes after the argument has subsided. Sometimes, telling your partner exactly what you just read here can ignite a loving spark in them and lead you into the most meaningful conversation that manages to get a lot of things sorted out.

Seeking Help

As mentioned earlier, there is always the option of getting a third party involved and seeking counsel or guidance with them. Friends and family can be an indispensable source of support in these difficult situations. In fact, talking to a friend or trusted family member isn't some last-ditch option that should only be used if all else fails. There's nothing wrong with turning to a friend early on.

Of course, it is okay if you prefer to solve these problems without bringing anyone into the story, but you should know that no friend or loved one will think less of you for discussing the things that bother you. Don't be constrained by notions of pride, manhood, or any other inhibitor preventing you from opening up. This is what friends and family are for. If you feel your relationship is in jeopardy, go seek advice that applies to your specific situation.

However, when you bring other people into the problem, you must make sure that you give them a clear and objective picture of the situation that's bothering you. If they don't have the right idea of what's going on, the most well-intentioned of friends can become fountains of terrible advice and only make things worse. If possible, it might be best for you and your significant other to talk to friends or family together.

You must also make sure that your friends really are friends, of course. You have to be absolutely positive that you trust them before confiding in them about the problems going on in an important personal relationship. If the problem is serious, it might not be a good idea to ask mere acquaintances for advice. People can indeed have all sorts of ulterior motives in mind.

There is, however, a particularly bad stage that some dysfunctional relationships can reach where you absolutely have to look for help. I'm talking about abusive relationships, of course. If your husband, boyfriend, or another close person is violent toward you or terrorizes you psychologically on a daily basis, then it's time to confide in someone.

The fact that you don't sleep well due to constantly being traumatized is the least of the problems in such a relationship. If you're a victim of domestic violence, usually the best thing to do is look for help from the authorities. If you're unsure whether the situation is severe enough to call the police, a friend who cares about you can help you make that decision.

This should go without saying, but men too can be victims of domestic abuse. Even though the incidence of such cases is much lower than when the genders are reversed, the cases can still be severe or even deadly. If you're a man and something like this has happened, you have to fight through your pride or shame if your instincts are telling you that what's happening is wrong or dangerous.

At any rate, something else that you should consider for other, more civilized relationship problems is counseling. It really is unfortunate that married couples can get to a point where they can't communicate effectively enough to solve their own problems, but that's just how life is sometimes. Marriage counseling can be highly beneficial both in support groups and with individual professionals and therapists.

Fighting for a relationship with someone whom you truly love and care about is a noble cause and is always worth the trouble. There are limits, however, particularly to the length of time that you should devote to someone who constantly disappoints you, betrays you, and just does you wrong at every turn. There comes a time when you have to ask yourself if you've done all you could and if it's time to quit for your own sake.

As difficult as it can be to admit, the truth is that a certain, small percentage of people are beyond help. The relationships with them can become a waste of valuable emotional resources and precious time, which often turns into years. Indeed, some relations are unfixable, whether they are romantic, familial, or friendships. It can appear unthinkable, especially when it's a family member, but these things do happen. I have no way of telling if you happen to be in such a relationship. The answer to that question is in your heart if you care to look hard enough.

In these cases, the only solution left in the end is to let go. This is where a true and trusted friend can be perhaps the most helpful because making this decision on your own can be the hardest thing, even impossible. You should never underestimate your capacity for blindness when it comes to the people you love or used to love. These deep, long-standing feelings can completely impair our judgment, which is why a friend should come in and give us a reality check.

Even after we manage to let go, a prolonged period of adjustment might ensue, resulting in recurring dreams, restless nights, outbursts of heavy thoughts, and much else. Out of sight does indeed mean out of mind, though, at least on a long enough timeline. In the end, you will learn to go on without the toxic figures of the past; they will seem as little more than a bad dream you once had, and you will sleep easy again.

Chapter Twelve: Seek Professional Assistance

Based on the long talk we've just had, one thing should be especially apparent: treating your insomnia more or less translates to an effort to tidy-up your life. Indeed, our sleeping pattern can perhaps be viewed as a reflection of how we live our life. A messy and unhealthy lifestyle tends to cause messy and unhealthy sleep. Instead of responding only to the symptoms, the idea is to address every underlying cause, and those causes are often to be found outside your bedroom, though not always.

At any rate, if you find it difficult to implement these strategies and information or, by some miracle, none of it applies to you, seeking professional assistance is always another option on the table. As opposed to strolling into a psychiatrist's office for a quick prescription to suppress your symptoms artificially, which they will likely and happily provide, there are other options to consider.

Chronic insomniacs that have tried everything else usually turn to therapists and consultants, both in person and online, who have a wide range of approaches and programs for their patients. Although sleep coaching is my profession, don't get the idea that this is an advertisement. In this chapter, we will take a look at how insomnia is generally treated nowadays in the mainstream and go into a bit more detail about some of the techniques. In the event that you do decide to seek professional assistance for your insomnia, this information will help get you started on that path.

Insomnia Treatment Today

So, what does the "market" look like nowadays? We mentioned early on that the market relating to insomnia is expected to be worth some $4 billion just two years from now. While insomnia-related products such as pharmaceuticals certainly account for a big slice of that market, a lot of it is still made up of various forms of therapy. Some of these therapy techniques are more main-stream than others, but studies and patients have reported results from a wide range of different approaches.

The approach to insomnia treatment has evolved with our understanding of the disorder, of course, but the biggest shift perhaps occurred in recent decades. This is because insomnia used to be regarded as nothing but a mere symptom, always of a different medical condition, another sleep disorder, mental illness, and other similar problems. Of course, all of these things can cause insomnia, and insomnia is indeed often indicative of a larger problem, as you have learned.

However, chronic insomnia is definitely a disorder in and of itself. Another relatively recent revelation is everything we've talked about in this book in regard to behavior. We now know that insomnia can be and usually is a consequence of poor habits and life choices. Another problem for the older school of thought is that, in the event of a medical condition being the cause, insomnia can sometimes persist even after that condition has been cured. This potential for independence and the apparent insomnia epidemic happening nowadays have made experts all over the world take this condition much more seriously than previous generations.

The treatment of insomnia in the developed world generally takes one of three approaches: behavioral therapy, medication, or a combination of both. What you've been reading throughout this book is generally the behavioral therapy approach, focusing on eliminating problem behaviors and altering habits to fight insomnia. This field includes many sleep coaches and experts such as yours truly, many of whom can have their own unique approaches to treatment. There are also widely known and well-established programs such as cognitive behavioral therapy for insomnia (CBT-I), which we mentioned on a few occasions in this book. We will take a better look at this method soon.

Medical treatment for insomnia is self-explanatory. The third, combined approach, however, can vary quite a bit. Such a treatment technique can in many ways resemble what you've learned here, but with a higher tolerance for sleeping pills and other pharmaceuticals. Various exercises can be combined with occasional or short-term use of sleeping pills to assist the process, which can work very well, especially in less severe cases of insomnia.

These therapies can be taken at medical centers and other places that specialize in treating sleep disorders. Another venue is the Internet, of course, where you can find and follow therapy strategies such as this one or get some face time with an online therapist.

Overall, folks whose insomnia is particularly severe or unique tend to benefit the most from real-life behavioral therapy. Talking to a living, breathing sleep coach can certainly make a world of difference in such cases. Some people also can't afford to spend months and months perfecting these techniques on their own and slowly working their way toward the first great results. An actual therapy session, especially if highly tailored and personalized, can perhaps speed up the process. Of course, the main issue is that it doesn't come free and, depending on where you go for your therapy, might not come cheap either.

Cognitive Behavioral Therapy for Insomnia

Behavioral therapies, in general, will provide you with a variable and holistic program just like the one in this book. Behavioral therapy is more-or-less an umbrella term that can include some or all of the following: relaxation, cognitive therapy, stimulus control, holistic approaches to sleep hygiene improvement, and much else.

In general, a behavioral therapy program can yield results after between six and ten sessions, in addition to an introduction to the basics. The process tends to be the fastest when the patient already has knowledge or experience in fighting insomnia through strategies such as those in this book. If you have been considering getting professional therapy for a while now, then this book can serve as the perfect gateway to help you get the most out of therapy.

Cognitive therapy, as its name suggests, focuses on an insomniac's thinking process. In particular, this is a term that refers to sessions where therapists help the patient overcome some of those vicious cycles of anxiety and worry that we explained earlier. One example is obsessive and negative thinking in relation to the patient's insomnia, which, as you know, only makes the problem worse.

Cognitive behavioral therapy for insomnia, or CBT-I, is an approach that makes use of some of the aforementioned strategies that fall under behavioral therapy. It's a proven therapy technique that uses a holistic approach to focus both on the mind and the body. The strategies we have outlined here come together to form a sort of CBT-I program.

The typical CBT-I program that you can enroll in will usually span a period of several weeks. The most basic program consists of eight or so sessions and begins with an educational introduction about the way sleep works to help the patient understand his or her goals better. The next two sessions will deal with stimulus control and sleep restriction methods. Two cognitive therapy sessions usually follow these and are themselves followed by a session that teaches the patient about sleep hygiene in detail. The basic CBT-I program often ends with a session that's organized based on the way that the therapy went for that particular patient.

Many CBT-I programs tend to be mostly educational in nature, which can be perfect for many insomniacs. Participants will usually be given a means of keeping logs of their progress and results. With consultation from the therapists, the patient's therapy can be adjusted and tailored to their needs if necessary. Some CBT-I experts will also infuse their sessions with specific exercise regimens that we mentioned earlier, such as aerobics, yoga, or meditation. When you are given the time and attention of an expert in person, such a holistic approach can undoubtedly change your life and rid you of insomnia forever.

Many studies have looked into the effectiveness of CBT-I and other similar methods over the years. Because of this, CBT-I has acquired a lot of credibility and stands as one of the most effective, drug-free therapy methods for defeating insomnia and improving your life overall while you're at it. The studies have found that CBT-I improves all facets and stages of the patient's sleep.

On average, CBT-I cuts sleep latency by 19 minutes and improves sleep efficiency by 10% after a basic program. Most importantly, these improvements were found to persist in the long-term, well after the patient was done with the treatment. Of course, that is assuming that the former insomniac doesn't completely revert to his old, unhealthy ways the day he leaves treatment. Just like the stuff we covered, the skills you can learn in CBT-I therapy are the knowledge that you will take with you forever, and that's perhaps the greatest value of the sessions.

Additional Tips

There are many other therapy techniques that might produce the best possible results for your particular case. Your main challenge will be to find a medical center or an expert therapist in your area. If you do find one, it can turn out to be one of the more expensive options, so there can be an economic obstacle to boot.

As we briefly mentioned, however, insomnia therapy can be taken over the Internet or over the phone. As a matter of fact, some studies have also looked into the effectiveness of phone and Internet-based CBT-I. While the findings were mostly self-reported and not particularly detailed, there was a significant consensus among the participants that these delivery methods had helped them. Digital and phone services can hardly compare to the real deal, though, but in the absence of all other options, it's certainly worth a try. Besides, the research comparing the two delivery methods is still lacking, so the difference is rather inconclusive.

It stands to reason that a personal interaction would be more effective, and in some ways, it is, such as in the treatment of anxiety and depression, for instance. This is unsurprising since both of these problems are highly responsive to human interaction.

Another option that might work wonders for some people is a full-time sleep coach or consultant. If you find a good, experienced sleep coach, you will essentially have the therapy come to you. These experts will often visit you and do a thorough inspection of your living environment, your problems as you describe them, and your habits and overall lifestyle.

He or she will evaluate all of these things and come up with the best possible program based on your personal parameters. This is a great way to get the most tailored, personalized experience possible and be given the most attention from the therapist. The most knowledgeable and experienced coaches might be very versatile in that they can train you in yoga and meditation while covering the other angles as well.

On top of that, a coach can give you pointers in regards to whether or not your mattress, pillow, and sheets are good for you. They will notice a whole lot of things in your immediate surroundings that might be hindering your ability to get a good night's rest. Of course, a sleep coach can be just as difficult to find as an insomnia treatment center.

When you decide to look for any of these services, your best bet is to get on your Internet browser and get searching for anybody and anything in your vicinity that might be an expert on these things. Remember that insomnia is a widespread problem, so there are bound to be relevant forums and other platforms on the Internet where you can get in contact with other people who are looking for the same thing.

Such platforms will also often contain valuable feedback about different institutions and sleep consultants if you do find them. Do note that sleep consultants can also acquire certificates to demonstrate their knowledge and skills, and the more successful ones will usually have websites, blogs, or social media pages. There are also numerous public websites that list sleep coaches in different countries, states, cities, et cetera. As such, sleep consultants are far from being some underground practitioners with shady backgrounds and intentions. The best among them will be very transparent and quite active online, just like a whole range of other personal trainers that millions of people hire every day.

Conclusion

When you have insomnia, your liberation from it should immediately become one of your top priorities in life. It can't be overstated how profoundly this affliction can affect all facets of your life. It is an obstacle between you and success, functional relationships, the fulfillment of ambition, physical health, mental health, and all that is good in life. One of the things that make insomnia particularly bad is that suffering from it for a long time can get you used to your condition. It can make you forget how life used to be, and this is a terribly hopeless place to find yourself in.

Nobody should have to get used to being tired, irritable, anxious, and physically weak all the time, and nobody should be denied their most basic right to a night of quality rest. Forgetting what it's like to sleep normally can be a major problem for motivation, so you should beware this pitfall. Soldiering on through failures and periods of feeling unmotivated will eventually prove to be one of the most important feats of your life. Once you have gotten rid of chronic insomnia, your whole outlook on life will change for the better.

You have now been acquainted with many different steps and approaches, which you will be able to use selectively or in unison. I have given you the answers, but you will know best which of these answers apply the most to you. Remember what you have learned, though, and try to use as much of this information as you can because it certainly won't hurt you.

Taking time in the evening to relax with music and channeling your thoughts into a journal is healthy in general, whether you are an insomniac or not. This goes for most if not all of the steps we have covered, as they are welcome additions to anyone's life. If you think back on what you have learned, you will see things like the removal of harmful substances, spending time outdoors, finding a purpose, improving your diet, dealing with troubled relationships the right way, and looking for help with other things that might be bothering you.

Of course, this book's primary purpose was to help you overcome your insomnia, but you have also gathered some useful life advice. Either way, the important thing is to begin as soon as possible and get into it for the long run. Start small the very next day and gradually introduce as many of the strategies as you can and stick to the instructions as closely as possible.

Another thing to keep in mind is that no matter how long it takes for the strategies to start producing results, the change in your sleep won't happen overnight. It will take a while for your body to adjust and begin reaping the benefits, and different folks will have different experiences. For instance, even when you get to a point where your sleep has become easier and uninterrupted, you still might not experience that full refreshment when waking up. With time and with patience, however, it's bound to come along.

You should also keep in mind the final strategy that we covered. If you have stuck with the other strategies for months and they somehow don't yield results, you might need personalized, direct counseling. There is no shame in that, and you shouldn't feel like a failure. Some cases of insomnia have been developed for so long and they can run so deep that personal guidance truly is necessary.

You might feel that an inability to deal with your problem personally somehow makes you inadequate or lesser, but insomnia is not a case of caffeine addiction or some other mild addiction that is to be beaten. In its worst form, insomnia truly is an illness, and contracting this illness is hardly ever our fault. Folks can suffer from insomnia because of traumatic situations that they ended up in, things that were done to them, the hardships of everyday life, and much else. All of these are external factors that we never ask for. You'll know best what's bothering you, and you need to find a way to convince yourself that you can't and won't let it weigh on you any longer.

In the end, the important thing is that you have taken away three major points from the whole conversation. Firstly, insomnia strikes everywhere and is a major concern for an already-large yet constantly growing number of people – you are not the only one and you are certainly not cursed in any way. The second important point is that you are not beyond help, far from it. There is a way out and, while reading through these lines and paragraphs, you have seen the many approaches that are available to you.

The last but perhaps most important takeaway is that, despite all the information I have provided and all the help that you can seek out, your success will ultimately boil down to you and your own commitment. Make no mistake, even if you seek counseling and therapy, that's still a choice and commitment that you have to make. And even when you begin therapy, you have to stay involved and willing to work toward the resolution.

Reading this book has also been a step that you took personally, and that demonstrates that you have at least the basic will to fight this battle. The fact that you're here shows awareness about the problem and a realization that you need to tackle it. It might not seem like a major step to you right now, but what matters is that you've taken in. All you have to do now is start taking those next steps and persevering through whatever comes.

Things that are worthwhile rarely come easy, so you must prepare yourself mentally for potential failures. Keep your focus on the objective, work the program, and never lose sight of your desire for a good night's rest.

Resources:

Chapter 1
https://www.webmd.com/sleep-disorders/features/can-music-help-me-sleep#1
https://www.webmd.com/sleep-disorders/features/can-music-help-me-sleep#2
https://www.brooklynbedding.com/blog/music-for-sleep-tips-for-insomnia/
https://www.azumio.com/blog/health/music-treats-insomnia
https://universityhealthnews.com/daily/sleep/does-music-help-you-sleep-how-to-help-insomnia-by-listening-to-music/
https://www.sleepfoundation.org/articles/can-music-help-you-calm-down-and-sleep-better

Chapter 2
https://www.medicalnewstoday.com/articles/320611.php
https://www.vice.com/en_us/article/qvm9g3/advice-anxiety-worrying-insomnia
https://www.health.com/health/condition-article/0,,20188959,00.html
https://www.verywellmind.com/how-should-i-deal-with-negative-emotions-3144603
https://www.psychologytoday.com/intl/blog/in-practice/201802/5-overarching-principles-coping-negative-emotions
https://medium.com/the-mission/research-reveals-how-to-deal-with-negative-emotions-e9b0c3f7a2fd
https://www.psycom.net/stress-vs-anxiety-difference
https://www.healthline.com/health/stress-and-anxiety

Chapter 3
https://www.health.harvard.edu/staying-healthy/too-early-to-get-up-too-late-to-get-back-to-sleep
https://insomniacoach.com/forums/topic/is-sleep-restriction-recommended-for-waking-up-early/

Chapter 4
https://www.sleepfoundation.org/insomnia/what-causes-insomnia
https://www.verywellhealth.com/how-does-smoking-cigarettes-affect-sleep-3014709
https://www.webmd.com/diet/qa/does-caffeine-cause-insomnia
https://www.sleepfoundation.org/articles/caffeine-and-sleep
https://www.alcoholrehabguide.org/resources/dual-diagnosis/alcohol-and-insomnia/
https://www.sleepstation.org.uk/articles/insomnia/sleep-alcohol-and-mindful-drinking/
https://www.drinkaware.co.uk/alcohol-facts/health-effects-of-alcohol/effects-on-the-body/alcohol-and-sleep/
https://time.com/5414015/sleeping-pill-health-risks/
https://www.henryford.com/blog/2018/01/truth-sleeping-pills

Chapter 5
https://www.webmd.com/sleep-disorders/news/20100917/exercise-helps-you-sleep#1
https://www.sleepfoundation.org/articles/how-does-exercise-help-those-chronic-insomnia

https://www.yogajournal.com/poses/yoga-by-benefit/insomnia

https://www.sleepfoundation.org/articles/connection-between-yoga-and-better-sleep

https://www.telegraph.co.uk/news/health/7941641/Walking-to-a-good-nights-sleep.html

https://bottomlineinc.com/health/insomnia/walking-plan-to-stop-insomnia

https://www.iamyiam.com/blog/article/afternoon.walk.to.beat.insomnia

https://www.psychologytoday.com/us/blog/sleep-newzzz/201210/yoga-can-help-insomnia

Chapter 6

https://www.iamyiam.com/blog/article/afternoon.walk.to.beat.insomnia

https://www.health.com/sleep/falling-asleep-tv-on

https://www.clinicaladvisor.com/home/the-waiting-room/binge-watching-tv-and-its-effects-on-sleep/

https://edition.cnn.com/2016/11/09/health/smartphones-harm-sleep/index.html

https://www.independent.co.uk/life-style/health-and-families/health-news/mobile-phone-radiation-wrecks-your-sleep-771262.html

https://www.cnet.com/how-to/stop-your-gadgets-from-keeping-you-awake-at-night/

https://www.sleepfoundation.org/articles/how-meditation-can-treat-insomnia

https://eocinstitute.org/meditation/meditation-for-insomnia-and-better-sleep/

https://www.medicaldaily.com/life-hack-sleep-4-7-8-breathing-exercise-will-supposedly-put-you-sleep-just-60-332122

Chapter 7
https://www.sciencedaily.com/releases/2017/07/170710091734.htm
https://www.lexiyoga.com/discovering-your-lifes-purpose-cures-insomnia
https://www.theschooloflife.com/thebookoflife/insomnia-matters/
https://www.medicalnewstoday.com/articles/318406.php
https://thehumblepenny.com/the-power-of-generosity-and-why-it-pays
https://www.healthcentral.com/article/how-to-avoid-shiftwork-sleep-disorder
https://www.medicalnewstoday.com/articles/318377.php

Chapter 8
https://www.health.harvard.edu/staying-healthy/insomnia-restoring-restful-sleep
https://www.sleepfoundation.org/insomnia/symptoms/sleep-tips-insomnia-sufferers
https://www.verywellhealth.com/how-do-naps-affect-sleep-at-night-3014731
https://www.bustle.com/p/7-times-you-should-never-take-a-nap-no-matter-what-67601

Chapter 9
https://www.webmd.com/sleep-disorders/features/food-sabotage-sleep#1
https://www.aarp.org/health/healthy-living/info-2014/foods-that-disrupt-sleep-photo.html#slide1
https://www.psychologytoday.com/gb/blog/diagnosis-diet/201607/these-5-foods-and-substances-can-cause-anxiety-and-insomnia
https://www.medicalnewstoday.com/articles/32

4295.php

https://www.alaskasleep.com/blog/foods-for-sleep-list-best-worst-foods-getting-sleep

https://www.healthline.com/nutrition/9-foods-to-help-you-sleep#section11

https://www.mirror.co.uk/lifestyle/health/your-insomnia-down-what-you-1919884

Chapter 10

https://www.huffingtonpost.co.uk/entry/why-orgasms-help-you-sleep_n_57ade964e4b007c36e4e4f15?guccounter=2

https://www.psychologytoday.com/intl/blog/the-truth-about-exercise-addiction/201808/the-connection-between-sex-and-sleep

https://www.healthcentral.com/article/could-masturbation-cure-your-insomnia

https://sleepjunkies.com/4-alternative-insomnia-hacks/

https://www.huffingtonpost.co.uk/entry/why-orgasms-help-you-sleep_n_57ade964e4b007c36e4e4f15?guccounter=2#gallery/55a5458ce4b0ecec71bd1cb9/2

Chapter 11

https://losangeleswestsidetherapy.com/2012/08/10/cure-insomnia-by-dealing-with-anger-and-relationship-stress/

https://www.ncbi.nlm.nih.gov/pmc/articles/PMC3674886/

https://www.whittierhospital.com/WHMC-Blog/2016/August/Insomnia-FAQ.aspx

https://www.lovepanky.com/love-couch/broken-heart/how-to-fix-a-broken-relationship

https://www.yourtango.com/experts/dr-randi-gunther/8-things-couples-can-do-to-fix-broken-relationship

Chapter 12

https://www.health.com/sleep/sleep-coach

https://www.tuck.com/sleep-consultants/

https://www.theinsomniaclinic.co.uk/

https://www.internationalsleep.org/find-a-consultant

https://www.mayoclinic.org/diseases-conditions/insomnia/in-depth/insomnia-treatment/art-20046677

https://www.sleepfoundation.org/articles/cognitive-behavioral-therapy-insomnia

https://www.sleepfoundation.org/insomnia/treatment

https://www.uptodate.com/contents/behavioral-and-pharmacologic-therapies-for-chronic-insomnia-in-adults

Made in the USA
Las Vegas, NV
28 September 2022